LIFE LIGHT

Other titles by Keith Foster, available from Sagax Publishing 47 Haymill Close, Greenford, Middlesex, UB6 8HL at £10.95 each:

*Perfume, Astrology and You*
This book is about health, wealth and sexual attraction. It deals exclusively with the language of instinct, the oldest system of communication in the world.

Every human being alive on the planet today uses this language subconsciously all the time, but most people are completely unaware of its existence. Our instincts dictate the formation of every relationship we enter into, and through these they govern the state of our health, our wealth and our degree of sexual success.

This book contains the key to the secret language of instinct and emotion. It shows you how to use this language properly to get the best out of every situation.

*Cool Cooking* (The regeneration diet)
This book tells the story of a remarkable breakthrough in the field of nutrition. It shows you how you can change your diet completely yet live on the same food you've always eaten! It details new gourmet recipes prepared and to be enjoyed in a totally new way, a way which will enable you to become much more healthy and vigorous while saving a small fortune each month on your food and power bills. This book is a must for every cook and for everyone interested in full good health. It contains many new recipes and new methods of preparation bound up in a completely new philosophy of living.

*The Golden Age A History of the Twelve Gods of the Zodiac*
The story of the origins of humankind. This book deals in detail with the persistent rumours of Gods on earth and explains an age-old system of global communication still available to the few "in the know" today. The knowledge in this book will alter your view of both religion and history — forever.
IT EXPLAINS THE MEANING OF LIFE!

*Earth The Song Flower*
How Life Began And Developed On This Planet and where it's going
An easy to understand scientific explanation as to how the movement of the solar and stellar bodies affects life on earth. This book tells how we are all influenced by the subtle electromagnetic forces around us and it contains new and vital information on how these forces affect your health, sexuality and wealth.
IT SHOWS YOU HOW TO INFLUENCE YOUR FUTURE BY LEARNING TO MANIPULATE THE FIFTH DIMENSION.

# LIFE LIGHT

## HOW TO PROTECT YOURSELF FROM CANCER
*OR HELP YOURSELF IF YOU GET ILL*

KEITH FOSTER

SAGAX PUBLISHING
1998

Published by Sagax Publishing
Sagax Publishing
46 Haymill Close
Greenford
Mddx UB6 8HL

Copyright © Keith Foster 1997

ISBN 0 9532407-1-1

A catalogue record for this book is available from the British Library

Keith Foster's right to be identified as the author of this work has been asserted by him in accordance with the Copyright, Designs and Patents Act 1988.

Typeset in Palatino 12/13pt from the author's disk by Scriptmate Editions

Manufacture coordinated in UK by
Book-in-Hand Ltd, 20 Shepherds Hill, London N6 5AH

All rights reserved. No part of this book may be reproduced or transmitted in any form, electronic or mechanical, including photocopy or any information storage and retrieval system, without permission in writing from the publisher.

I dedicate this book to Colin Leonard,
who is an inspiration to the oppressed
and a friend to those in need.
A truly good man and a gifted healer.

## Foreword

I have known Keith Foster for a number of years and we have always shared a great interest in 'life, the universe and everything' and its meanings.

He has written an immensely interesting, informative and succinct book which has given me a great deal of food for thought. He combines considerable knowledge with some rare insights to produce a work which will greatly enhance the reader's understanding of the underlying mechanics of life itself, and allow an increased access to health and vitality. The layout is easy to follow, and the unfolding of information is fascinating.

His work on the nature of time is extremely thought-provoking and his perceptions truly enlightening in their connotations.

This book also provides considerable insight into geopathic and emotional stress and gives some unconventional and extremely useful solutions to these problems.

Altogether a stimulating and informative work.

Christopher M. Eedy D.O.
M.Cr.O.A., L.C.S.P(Phys), J.O.A., I.C.A.K(E).

## Introduction

Disease is the way that nature removes all organisms that are no longer healthy or viable in her scheme of things and which stand in the path of evolutionary progress.

The knowledge in this book is set out in such a way as to show you how to adjust your life so as to become healthy and viable again.

It is written in thoughtbyte form for ease of assimilation and is fully supported by the scientific evidence laid out in the works in the bibliography. The conclusions reached on the basis of these researches are my own and are based on my own observations and insights.

The theories and formulas presented in this book are expressed as my opinion and as such are not meant to be used to diagnose, prescribe, or to administer in any manner to any physical ailments. In any matters related to your health, please contact a qualified, licensed health practitioner (and ask them to arm themselves with a copy of this book so that you can work together to re-establish your health).

Caduceus symbol on front cover reproduced from *The Sun and The Serpent*, Hamish Miller & Paul Broadhurst, by kind permission of the publishers, Pendragon Press, Launceston, Cornwall.

Figure 4 reproduced from Lawrence Edwards, *The Vortex of Life*, by kind permission of the publishers, Floris Books, Edinburgh.

Figures 1, 3, 5 and 6 reproduced from Victor Schauberger (translated & edited by Callum Coates), *Living Energies*, by kind permission of the publishers, Gateway Books, Bath, Somerset.

## Contents

### CHAPTER ONE — 15
#### CANCER IS A DARK STATE OF LIFE

SPIRALS—GOD'S VOICE UPON THE WATERS—FERMENTATION—THE BEGINNING OF THE FLOW—THE BLOOM—MEMORY—COLOUR—LET THERE BE LIGHT—ENERGY—THE TRANSFORMATION—VITAMIN C—ELECTRON TRANSPORT—DARK LIFE—MITOSIS—FREE ENERGY—GENE CONTROL—ELECTRO-CHEMICAL LIFE—THE BATTERY—THE PROTECTIVE FIELD—CELL DIVISION—DIVIDE OR DIE—ELECTRON OUTFLOW—FLAT BATTERY—THE THROWBACK—CELLULAR POTENTIAL/CHARGE

### CHAPTER TWO — 25
#### THE HUMAN 'PATTERN'

CELL COOPERATIVES—SUB-SYSTEMS—THE SIGNAL—THE COMMUNICATION—THE BRAIN—GLIAL CELLS—MOBILITY—POWER USE—POWER SUPPLY—THE TRANSCEIVER—SEPARATE SIGNALS—ABERRANT TRANSMISSIONS—THE MECHANISM—RED BLOOD CELLS—LOW FREQUENCY CURRENT—WHITE BLOOD CELLS—THE REGULATOR—THE RECHARGE SYSTEM—UNSTABLE STATES—THE DEGREE OF RESPONSE—EMOTIONAL STRESS—POWER LOSS—TRANSLOCATED GENES—SHOCK OR HYPER-IRRITATION—THE COHERENT GENE—THE SEVEN TONES—ASYMMETRY—THE ELECTRO-IMMUNE SYSTEM—SPINS—THE HYPERFINE INTERACTION—SPIN REVERSAL

### CHAPTER THREE — 38
#### HEALTH POWER

STRESS—WHERE POWER COMES FROM—VORTICES—PULSATION—THE SECOND LAW OF THERMO-DYNAMICS—NATURE—SPIRAL HELICAL STRUCTURES—THE ENERGY SPIRAL—CENTRIPETAL FORCE—BLOOD CIRCULATION—CELLULAR RECHARGE—HEART BEAT—BACTERIA, HEAT AND CO2—SUMMARY—ACTIVE AIR—INTENTIONAL IONS—PLANT GROWTH—AIR CONDUCTIVITY—POWER LEACHING AIR—WITCH WINDS—THUNDER STORMS, LIGHTNING AND RAIN—SPIRAL BREATHING

### CHAPTER FOUR — 54
#### THE LATTICE OF LIFE

THE MAGNETOSPHERE—BOW WAVE—SEVEN DRUMS—THE CHORD—PATTERNS OF RHYTHMIC ACTIVITY—THE FLOW—THE MOON—THE LUNAR PUMP—THE PATHWAYS—THE DOUBLE HELIX CONTRA-FLOW OF POWER—ACUPUNCTURE—MERIDIANS—RADIOACTIVE PHOTOGRAPHY

## CHAPTER FIVE 62
### WATER ENERGY

CLATHRATE SUBSTANCES—MICRO-STRUCTURES—ELECTROLYSIS—PROPERTIES—ENERGY—SPECIFIC-HEAT CURVE—VIBRATIONS—MEMORY—MOVEMENT AND SPACE—PROPORTIONS—HARMONY—RESONANCE

## CHAPTER SIX 71
### FOOD ENERGY

THE FORCE OF LIFE—VITAL RESERVES—DEAD FOOD—THE FOOD CHAIN—THE DOUGHNUT—THE CATABOLIC RATE—THE 'NUB' OF NUTRITION—LEUKOCYTOSIS (Increased White Blood Cell Count)—INCREASED ENZYME COUNT—COOKED FOOD—FEAST AND FAMINE—KIRLIAN PHOTOGRAPHY (Electro-luminescent discharge from organisms)—OUR TRUE LIFE SPAN—QUANTITY VERSUS QUALITY

## CHAPTER SEVEN 79
### ELECTRICITY, MAGNETISM AND ELECTROMAGNETIC ENERGY

EARTH'S FIELDS—SUPER-CONDUCTOR—COHERENCE AND CHAOS—MAJOR SYSTEMS—THE TRANSFORMATION—CHIRAL FORMS—NORTH-SOUTH POLARITY—ORGANIC POLARITY—WHAT COMES NEXT—OUR NEW ELECTROMAGNETIC ENVIRONMENT—UNNATURAL FIELDS—DNA OSCILLATORS—ENTRAINMENT—HOMEO-DYNAMICS—UNNATURAL COHERENT INFLUENCES—ULTIMATE STABILITY—SUMMARY

## CHAPTER EIGHT 90
### MIND

MOODS—THE MIND-BRAIN-ENZYMIC RELATIONSHIP—TWO CENTRES—THE SOLAR PLEXUS—UNITY AND FOCUS—HARMONY—THE BALANCE—THE FLOW—PATHCURVES—THE CREATION OF ENERGY—INTERLOCKING VORTICES—LIVING ENERGIES—TIME—CAUSE AND EFFECT?—PHYSICAL FORM—TWO VORTEX—TWIN CONES—TWO POLES—THE PHYSICAL BODY—CONSCIOUS CONTROL—THE PURPOSE OF LIFE—SINGLE CURVES—LEARNED EVENTS—THE HUNDREDTH MONKEY SYNDROME

### CHAPTER NINE — 108
### WHAT TO DO TO HELP YOURSELF

THE BEGINNING—VITAMIN C—HEALING CRISIS—PREFERRED FORMS—OVEREATING—FOOD STRESS—THE POISON INDUSTRY—JUICING—ADJUSTMENTS—DIET—A SACCULATED BOWEL—FASTING—COOL COOKING—FLAVOURS—TASTE—SHOOTS—MONEY—AIR—REAL AEROBIC EXERCISE

### CHAPTER TEN — 131
### CONCLUSION

WATER—HEALTHY WATER—WATER-BORNE DISEASES—IMPURITIES—THE WRONG SPIN—DISSOLVED MINERALS—RIPE WATER—REMOVING ELECTROMAGNETIC POLLUTION FROM WATER—REMOVING CHEMICAL POLLUTION FROM WATER—LEFT-HAND RIGHT-HAND—AMPHORA—NATURE'S COOLERS—ROCK MEAL—SINGING SAND—PROTECTING YOURSELF FROM ELECTROMAGNETIC FIELD EFFECTS—COPPER WIRE—THE SOLUTION—EXORCISING STRESS—EMOTIONAL STRESS—DOMINANT MENTAL STATE—HOW TO CHANGE YOUR DOMINANT MENTAL ATTITUDE—ANGER—GROWING—YOUR GROWTH—CHANGE—NEW DIRECTIONS—REPROGRAMMING—THE FLOW—FINAL PRACTICALITIES

### BIBLIOGRAPHY — 155

### PRODUCT INDEX — 157

# CHAPTER ONE

## CANCER IS A DARK STATE OF LIFE

Three billion years ago when the earth was still hot and covered by an atmosphere thick with dust and smoke — dark life began. As the surface of our planet began to cool water formed in the atmosphere and rocks and it started to rain. Over millions of years the rain dissolved chemicals from the dust and gases in the atmosphere, collecting in large lagoons in the still hot earth below.

The first building blocks of dark life were crude amino-acids formed in the primeval sea. We can reproduce this "first step" in the laboratory today by splashing chemical mixtures dissolved in water on to hot rocks. But way back then the life force had a whole planet to work with.

As time passed, clumps of these fatty acids were swept together by the storm wind and tides to form dense concentrations in the warm shallow seas.

### SPIRALS

At that time the earth's atmosphere was still dark and turbulent. Huge electrical storms raged across the face of the earth blasting millions of volts of lightning into the seas beneath. The energy from these lightning volts fizzed outward from the point of impact forming bush-shaped clumps of spirals in the thicker watery medium.

The spiral forms the template of all life. Everything moves in spirals because the shortest distance between two moving objects isn't a straight line as you would expect, but is in fact a spiral.

As time went by this spiral energy input caused the concentrations of amino-acids to string together into molecules of protein, the most fundamental chemical ingredient in the development of a dark-life form.

## GOD'S VOICE UPON THE WATERS

The vast storms ultimately settled into a complex pattern of weather fronts which were self-similar. This self-similarity is called a fractal form, and simply means that they fall into an orderly pattern out of the original chaos.

The extremely low frequency but rhythmic rolling thunder of the storm fronts shook the waters of the deep causing the proteins to clump into organic patterns.

In time these patterns of protein began to behave cooperatively and the first complex structures of dark life were born.

At first these were not true cells as we know them today, but simply micro-organisms whose cellular contents were not bound by distinct membranes. They were basically blobs of jelly with nucleic material spread throughout the blob.

## FERMENTATION

It was still dark on the surface of the earth and these early dark-life forms were not very active because there was not much energy available for them to use. Nevertheless, as yet more millions of years passed, these first flickerings of dark life learnt to use every source of energy available to them, including electricity.

During this period they developed fermentation as their main power source, fermenting sugar-like molecules from their environment for energy.

## THE BEGINNING OF THE FLOW

For any life activity there has to be an energy flow, and to have an energy flow there has to be a mechanism which enables it to flow.

The problem that faced our early protein ancestors was that they were made out of relatively large, clumsy macromolecules in which the electrons were held firmly in their orbits and have no mobility.

Electrons are the small negatively charged electric particles that surround the atomic core of a molecule, and to have a flow of energy these have to move from molecule to molecule. This is called electron transport.

This situation is best illustrated by a full parking lot, nothing can move until one car is taken out, and then all the rest can move (but not much).

The only electron conductor/acceptor available to early dark life was a weak chemical mixture called methyl-glyoxal. This couldn't conduct energy very well but when attached to the proteins it was a start, and dark life quickly cashed-in on this advantage by beginning to form proper cells with cell walls and nuclei.

THE BLOOM

Algae bloomed into dark life and formed into a fabulous wealth of different types, each capable of eking out a living from next to nothing, by converting all the available energy to their use. The early algae manufactured multiple sugars and used these to build the cellulose containers around themselves which we know today as cell walls. These cells were capable of reproducing themselves.

More than three thousand million years ago they developed every form of asexual and sexual reproduction known throughout the entire plant and animal world today. They reproduce themselves in their multi-millions by simple fission (splitting), budding (like yeast), fragmentation (breaking in bits) and most important of all to us — by mitosis — (complex division).

MEMORY

The nucleus of each cell usually contains genes which are the memory banks of the cell. These are the store-house of the accumulated experience of the cell and are used to direct all its functions. Genes are made up of the chemical spiral deoxyribonucleic acid (DNA) and they are all organised as strands called chromosomes. Every cell alive today remembers every step in its long long evolutionary history, through its genes, and these genes, as we shall see later, have a lot to do with cancer.

### COLOUR

As the algae bloomed, specialised and proliferated, it took on different colours from its surroundings. These colours were all part of its scavenging for energy but were to prove spectacularly successful in dark life's great leap forward.

### LET THERE BE LIGHT

For millions of years it had rained. Huge torrents of liquid titrated from the atmosphere and pounded down on the ever cooling earth bringing with them billions of tons of dust. As the sky's cleared light could penetrate to the surface and light life as we know it began.

Light is made up of photons which are small parcels of energy sliding along a wave, like brightly lit beads on a string. This energy input was a God-send to life on earth as it separated the elements of water into hydrogen and oxygen. This liberated oxygen, which has a net negative charge, to act as the best possible electron acceptor/conductor and vital to light life, as we shall see.

At last the life force had the power to flow and began to develop the mechanism to use the power.

### ENERGY

The algae rapidly learnt to absorb and use this new energy source. Different coloured algae absorbed or reflected different colours out of the light. The rate of absorption dictated the rate at which they were able to synthesise carbon dioxide and water. A waste product of this carbon fixation process was more oxygen.

The visible light spectrum rises from red through orange, yellow, green, blue, purple to indigo. So that the blue light higher up the spectrum has more energy than the red light at the bottom. Because of this blue-green algae were able to gain an advantage over the other types and evolved ever more complex structures.

They developed chlorophyll as their main energy conversion mechanism and their various component colours became the first vitamins, enzymes and co-enzymes.

Enzymes and co-enzymes govern or regulate cellular activity starting and stopping, speeding up or slowing down reactions. Vitamins on the other hand are essential for normal cell function, the actual work of a cell, and the most important of these is vitamin C — as we shall see.

### THE TRANSFORMATION

Back down amongst the clumsy protein molecules an even more revolutionary transformation was taking shape. The blocked up parking lot had suddenly emptied, leaving the few remaining cars to whiz around in a highly active state. What had happened was that vitamin C and oxygen had come together to provide life's flow mechanism.

### VITAMIN C

Vitamin C is essential to the mechanism of life because it can easily pass one of its electrons to oxygen. When it does this its remaining structure becomes destabilised and is known as a very reactive free radical. This is a molecule that's lost an electron and needs to absorb another as quickly as possible to get back into balance. It does this by taking an electron from the methyl-glyoxal attached to the protein. By doing this it enables the protein to pass more electrons down this chain to the oxygen.

So that in the light-living state the protein molecules have plenty of space to move around — a high level of electronic activity.

### ELECTRON TRANSPORT

This bridge from the protein to the methyl-glyoxal to the vitamin C to oxygen, is basic to most life on this planet, and acts both as a bridge and an essential buffer. If oxygen could take electrons straight from protein we'd burn up in a rapid oxidation. As it is, it is a regulated process requiring lots of vitamin C.

Vitamin C transducing the protein into the living state enables it to perform. The more vitamin C available the better the protein will work.

### DARK LIFE

In the early period of life before light, only simple organisms could be built to perform only the simplest reactions. The most important of these actions was proliferation and this was helped by the simplicity of cell structures. All they had to do was replicate and replicate and replicate again, in an unending series of divisions until all the available nutrients were used up. This did not use much energy but was a very strong process indeed, because although the large protein molecules are not very active, when they did bond, the cohesive forces that held them together were the strongest living forces then available.

After light life developed however, cell structures became increasingly complex and capable of much more varied, more organised cooperation. They organised into a vast variety of life forms, each made up of a host of co-operating cellular colonies held together by a common purpose. However, each cell "remembered" its ancestry in its genetic code.

### BONDS

Because light driven reactions are so much more energy rich, the forces that bind them together are far more vital than the dark driven fermentation reactions. But they only work properly when lots of energy is available. If the energy is not available then the cells will ultimately snap back into the dark life fermentation mode for their energy supply.

### MITOSIS

Structures and cohesion interfere with cell division because their purpose is to hold everything together, so when a light-driven cell divides it has to drop its structural defences and relax its binding cohesive forces — it has to return to the dark state!

Usually the two daughter cells of mitotic division will reform into the light state again. But if there isn't enough energy available to them they will get stuck in the dark state which we call cancer.

### FREE ENERGY

All the energy used by light life comes ultimately from the sun. The sun's energy drives photosynthesis in green plants which form organic molecules from the minerals in the earth and the gases in the atmosphere. Animals in turn get their energy by eating these plants and converting the molecules into energy they can use. The final receiving and processing "power-house" of this energy is the cell.

### GENE CONTROL

Cells have become very sophisticated and advanced structures since their early dark life beginnings. They have added billions of years of experience into their genetic structures, and now these genes control a wide range of sophisticated functions. All these functions require energy, and this energy is what dictates all cellular activity.

### ELECTRO-CHEMICAL LIFE

It's common to think of the human body as being a purely chemical structure, but this is obviously not the case. It is, in fact, an electro-chemical structure where the electrical reactions occur at an atomic level and are later amplified by the cruder chemical responses. Light life from the sun drives a series of basically chemical mechanisms which ultimately end up as stored electrical energy in the cell.

### THE BATTERY

Electrical energy is stored in a number of complex chemicals in the cell. The best known of these chemical reactions is phosphorylation where energy is stored in adenosine triphosphate (ATP). This is the final stage in a mechanism life has developed by which nutrients with different chemical and electrical structures are absorbed from the blood and the surrounding environment. These are then processed into ever more complex chemicals with more "concentrated" electrical charges and stored for future use. These chemicals with their different electrical properties are used by the cell in all its functions. This is the cells power supply and is basically a battery or accumulator which stores electrons.

THE PROTECTIVE FIELD

Electrons as we know are negatively charged particles from the outer shell of a molecule. (A bit like planets from around the sun). And it is because of these concentrations of electrons that a healthy cell normally has a strong negative charge. This negative charge creates a negatively charged electromagnetic field around the cell. This field is able to detect and inter-react with other fields and other charges in its vicinity. It can't be stable because it reacts continually to the electronic balance within the cell, as well as to the fields of the other cells around it.

CELL DIVISION

When cells divide as we have seen they do so in response to stress. The stress can be a physical blow, a chemical poison, an electromagnetic shock, a too high level of radiation, a thermal shock, an emotional shock (which gives rise to dangerous levels of neuro-hormones in the blood), or one of many other stressors. The important point though is that the stressor must be of an order of magnitude large enough to overcome the cells protective field. Normally a cell will ride out a shock by passing it on to the cells around it. The shock "wave" passes through the structure of the body causing some changes but doing little permanent harm.

### DIVIDE OR DIE

But if the shock is big enough to override the cells ability to "pass it on" then the cell must either divide or die. Usually the cell will divide by temporarily dropping its defences which flicks it back into the dark life state and reforming as two daughter cells (in light life again). During its brief dark life phase its genes instruct its "battery" to deliver enough energy to reform as two daughter cells, and all goes well. It re-emerges restructured as two light life cells. The problem is that the mechanism of stress response can be cumulative!

### ELECTRON OUTFLOW

When stressed the field around the cell reacts to the stress either by passing it on to the cells around it or by division as we've seen. Either way it uses energy. Electrons flow out of the cell in response to the stress, which causes a reduction in the power balance in the cell. Its "battery" is drained by the amount of energy used.

### FLAT BATTERY

If the cell isn't stressed again for some time its "battery" will recharge. But if the energy drain is high, with constant stresses, then the battery flattens. It runs out of power! When the cell's power falls to a low level of energy its defensive shield fades. With reduced defences it becomes sensitive to lower levels of stressor, and the next stress that overwhelms its defences, causes it to divide or die. At the level where it still has enough energy left to divide in response to stress, it switches into dark life. Exhausted by stress and continual division the cell has little power. It can't obey the genetic instructions developed during light life. These require a higher power level than is left in the cell. Its "read out" apparatus which is called the RNA, can only hunt downwards to lower power level instructions. It goes back in time to the earlier dark life instructions on the early part of the chromosome.

## THE THROWBACK

When these earlier genes order the reconstruction at the lower power level, the two daughter cells form as always, but this time they're cancerous! They are programmed to replicate, replicate, replicate. To ferment for energy, rather than getting it from the light driven reactions of normal cellular life. They now have to leach nutrients from their environment to fuel their reactions. Their defensive field is very weak because there isn't much electronic activity going on within the cell. With a low defence threshold they are prey to every stressor. Their fermentation driven reactions, using few electrons give them a very low level of electronic charge and they are therefore able to attract and bond to other cells around them which may be suffering also from charged depletion. Their polarity is much weaker. (Remember like charges repel unlike charges attract).

## CELLULAR POTENTIAL/CHARGE

Whilst they are cancerous or in the dark life state, cells have a lower level of electronic activity, they are fermenting nutrients for their energy supply. This is a strong reaction but not a very vital one and relative to the cells around them (which are getting their charge from the light driven reaction) dark life cells have a lower level of charge. (This is why all tumours have a lower electrical potential than healthy tissue). Healthy cells have a net negative charge because their light driven reactions can "pack in" more electrons. Electrons are negatively charged entities and as a cell the more you can store the higher your negative charge will be.

Cancerous cells being more positively charged than healthy cells are attracted to healthy cells very strongly and when they lock onto them perform the cellular equivalent of grand larceny leaching out all of their nutrients and redistributing their electronic charge thus causing them to flick into the dark life state also. This is one of the main reasons that cancers can grow so quickly.

## CHAPTER TWO

## *THE HUMAN 'PATTERN'*

When life first stirs in the human embryo it has a particular pattern of energy. This pattern derives from its spiral DNA which is the result of the "chance" combination of different series of genes from the parents' chromosomes. This pattern in the DNA is unique to each individual. It dictates their exact growth and development down to the last structural detail. Down to the last skin blemish or grey hair. Every single cell in the human body contains identical DNA. Every single cell is capable of reproducing the entire overall pattern from this spiral code of genetic instructions.

### CELL COOPERATIVES

The human body is made up of a gigantic number of cells which all cooperate with each other. They are all basically separate individual cells. The instructions which tell them to cooperate together are located in genes which are placed very early on the chromosome. This cooperation began very early when cells were first formed into organic shapes by the thunder drum as we saw in Chapter One. The cells of each human body cooperate because they have the same identical code of instructions on their DNA. The DNA spiral behaves as an antenna or broadcast system telling each cell what to do.

### SUB-SYSTEMS

Within the body there are thousands of sub-systems or smaller cooperatives. These make up different organs or perform different functions. The cells of each of these organs differ from the cells of other organs. They are specific to each organ or system. However, all the cells in a body are basically the same. They have just adapted to perform a particular function. If a healthy cell is transplanted from one organ to another, it soon takes on the characteristics of the cells in the organ its placed on to. It conforms to that organ's signal.

### THE SIGNAL

Each system of the body is controlled by its own signal. So that all the cells in that cooperative know how to function. These signals are electromagnetically derived as we shall see.

### THE COMMUNICATION

Every system in the body depends on the cooperation of every other system in the body for survival. Information on the status of every organ/system in the body is passed from cell to cell throughout the entire body by the electron spin transfer process. This works like a bucket line of information going backwards and forwards to and from the brain. The information flows almost instantaneously to the brain which immediately sends back signals. These signals adjust each system's performance. The brain controls the entire body by continually receiving and broadcasting the overall DNA pattern. This is received and acted upon by the part or section of the DNA of each cell which regulates its specific cooperatives function.

### THE BRAIN

Contained within the bony protective casing of the skull, the brain looks like a large walnut kernel. This is because the more recently developed parts are wrapped around the older areas with lots of folds. The folds are there to give the newer area called the neo-cortex, a very large surface area in a smallish space. The brain is an electrically powered electricity generating organ of awesome complexity. It contains more neuron cells than there are stars in the universe, and each of these is as complex as a small computer. They produce and transmit electrical impulses. These travel from the cell body down along the fibres called axons until they reach another junction or synapse with another neuron cell. The electrical impulses fire chemical messengers called neuro-transmitters to receptors on the next cell. Because each neuron can be connected to thousands of other neurons, a single signal can electronically alter millions of other neurons. Each neuron is unique and has slightly different response patterns to all the others. Because of this the brain has billions of electromagnetic signals flying in all directions at all times. The neurons are fundamentally the "hard wired" system of the brain.

### GLIAL CELLS

As well as neurons the brain contains billions of glial cells which are ten times more numerous than the neurons. The glial cells are even more electrically sensitive than the neurons and unlike neurons, these can divide and become cancerous. Glial cells are like liquid crystals which resonate in harmony with the surrounding electromagnetic fields. By doing this they act like transistors picking up electrical impulses from the environment as well as from the neurons. They amplify these signals tens of thousands of times passing them on to the neurons. As we can see later, this extreme sensitivity to electromagnetic fields is now one of the main contributory factors leading to cancerous conditions.

### MOBILITY

Unlike neurons which are more or less fixed in position, the glial cells are extremely mobile. At times before the neurons sprout axons to connect with each other, the glial cells divide and actually move through the intact tissue of the brain. They migrate through large sections to get to a bio-electrically active site. Once there they send out branches and become very much bigger. This activity nourishes the surrounding fixed neurons and considerably increases the electrical capability of that part of the brain. This is what happens when we concentrate.

### POWER USE

The brain is primarily formed from one of the most unsaturated fats in the body. It is effectively a room temperature super-conductor because it has no electrical resistance. Although the brain is only 2 per cent of total body weight, it uses more than 20 per cent of all the oxygen taken into the body. Oxygen as we know has a negative charge and the brain is the most stupendous energy transformer in the body by far.

### POWER SUPPLY

During periods of great physical stress the heart diverts blood from other organs in order to supply the maximum available blood to the muscles and heart. The two organs bearing the greatest strain. But no matter what is going on at any time, the blood supply to the brain remains absolutely constant. It is the bodies main priority.

### THE TRANSCEIVER

The brain and spinal column (which is part of the brain) are bathed in a special fluid, rich in vitamin C. Vitamin C is natures best electron conductor/acceptor. There is 100 per cent more vitamin C in the cerebro-spinal fluid than in ordinary blood. This cushions the brain from shock and oxidation as well as providing a superb antenna for all the brain signals.

### SEPARATE SIGNALS

The identity signal of each cooperative of cells originates in the DNA. Each cooperative organ has a different signal. This is because each signal originates in a different part of the spiral antenna of the DNA. In this way liver cells receive and transmit liver cell instructions. Heart cells receive and transmit heart cell instructions and so on. All these signals are received at different levels of the spinal cord. The spinal cord transmits these signals instantly to the brain. The brain receives these different components of signals which altogether make up a complex code of fluctuating frequencies. The glial cells amplify this code which is then transmitted to the neuron cells. The neurons check and adjust the various signal strengths and frequencies. Then they rebroadcast the code correctly according to the overall DNA pattern. This is transmitted back via the spinal column, thence back to the various cooperatives or organs telling them what to do and how to do it.

### ABERRANT TRANSMISSIONS

Cells which are stressed into too rapid division, lose power as we have seen. As their power levels fall they switch into the dark life state. Here they ferment for energy. Fermentation does not deliver enough power for them to continue the information dialogue with the brain. As the recognition signals fail, the immune system can then take over and attack and destroy these aberrant cells. Similarly, if the brain continually gives off aberrant signals, then the weaker members of the cellular cooperative will respond to these. The cellular response is mediated by the energy level of the cell. As energy levels fall in response to stress the two-way process of information can go "out of tune" causing illness. Extreme cases of this signal failure become cancerous. The immune system deals basically with "self" and "not self" signals according to this mechanism.

### THE MECHANISM

A normally functioning immune system is an effective defence against foreign infectious agents and against body cells that have become cancerous. The immune regulatory mechanisms are genetically controlled. In humans these genes are located on the short arm of chromosome six. They regulate the different cellular components of the immune system, whose job it is to recognise and deal with foreign or damaged materials in the body. The main components of the immune system are different forms of blood cells and a complex of chemicals known as the complement cascade. Some blood cells originate in the bone marrow as what are called stem cells and become different types of blood cells as they pass into the bloodstream. White blood cells form the most active component of the immune system and represent only 1 per cent of the total blood volume. Red cells also play a role in the body's defence, although not as actively as the white cells.

All blood cells are manufactured in the bone marrow at the rate of 200 million a day.

### RED BLOOD CELLS

Red blood cells go straight into the circulatory system. They live there for about four months and travel around the body about 500,000 times a month. As they pass through the lungs, they absorb the negatively charged oxygen, transporting this through the body and delivering it to the cells. They then absorb the positively charged carbon dioxide released from the cells and let this out through the lungs again. Red blood cells are attracted to carbon dioxide about 200 times more than they are attracted to oxygen. Because of this they are very effective cleaning up agents in the bloodstream and an important part of the immune system.

### LOW FREQUENCY CURRENT

The blood circulation system basically provides a low frequency current carrying both positively and negatively charged particles to and from all the cells in the body. The cells use this power supply to perform their work.

### WHITE BLOOD CELLS

There are four main types of white blood cells produced by the bone marrow as stem cells. Two of these, called the macrophage and the granulocyte, circulate all the time in the bloodstream. These are the prowling predators of the immune system which can recognise and attack foreign or damaged cells. The mechanism they use to do this is electromagnetic as we shall see.

### THE REGULATOR

The other two types of white blood cells are called t-lymphocytes and b-lymphocytes. The b-lymphocyte cells distribute themselves around the body with the other two types and are effective in a complex reaction of all four types of white blood cells, which is controlled and mediated by the activity of the t-lymphocytes. Once t-lymphocytes become mature they migrate to the thymus gland. This is called a thymus because its discoverer thought it looked like a bunch of thyme. Because of their location of the thymus gland they're called t-lymphocytes, "t" for thymus. The thymus gland is part of the regulatory system of the body which is controlled by the mind, by mental states. It is the thymus acting in concert with the rest of the glandular system which regulates the immune system response.

## THE RECHARGE SYSTEM

As we've seen it is the job of the red cells to carry oxygen and nutrients to the cells, and to clean up the system by carrying waste products and carbon dioxide through the cleansing organs and lungs. During each cycle they pass electrons (particles having a negative charge) to the cells which use them and pass back positive charges to be disposed of. In this way the red blood cells perform a useful part of the immune function and often assist the white cells, as we shall see. It is the white cells that are the true "enemy killers" in the immune system. This is how they work:

> White cells circulating in the blood pass through the lungs in the same way as red cells. Whereas the red cells pick up a slight negative charge from the oxygen they absorb, the white cells pick up a very strong negative charge. The white blood cells absorb negative ions from the air. Negative ions, as we shall see later, are highly active oxygen molecules which have gained an electron. White cells carry these throughout the body where they play an important function in maintaining the body's energy levels. The bloodstream circulates throughout the body. There is no cell in the body more than a few cells away from a flow of blood. All the healthy cells in the body have a negative charge and a negative field around them. The white blood cells help maintain that charge by strengthening the polarity of the cells as they pass by. They reinforce the body's electronic structure and pass on, being repelled by healthy cell fields.

## UNSTABLE STATES

Cancer cells, bacteria and viruses all have differing electrical properties from normal cells. They are all unstable in low frequency currents such as the bloodstream. Consequently, the white blood cells are attracted to them. They home in on them being attracted by an opposite charge. They then multiply and cancel out the positive charges in the bacteria virus or cancer cell. By doing so they destroy themselves and the positive charge in the process. The debris is cleaned up by the red blood cells.

## THE DEGREE OF RESPONSE

The amount of activity the macrophage and b-lymphocyte white cell depends on the t-lymphocyte cells from the thymus. The t-lymphocyte cell matures in the thymus, receiving its final programming as part of that cooperative. It is genetically programmed within the cooperative. It learns there to be extremely responsive to the signals of neuro-hormones, as they affect that cooperative. When t-lymphocyte cells are mature, they travel into the spleen, lymph nodes and blood. Here they begin to perform the same as other white cells until stimulated into their attack mode. In the attack mode, they either amplify or suppress the activity of the other white blood cells. Their degree of activity and competence depends on the signals they are receiving from the thymus at that time.

## EMOTIONAL STRESS

The immune system is very sensitive to emotional and mental states. These dramatically alter the levels of stress neuro-hormones in the blood. Stress neuro-hormones effectively reduce the glial activity in the brain by concentrating glial activity into the more primitive response areas of the brain. This has the effect of directing the blood supply away from all the various organs in the body. They concentrate the blood supply in the heart, muscles and brain. This stress response starves the other organs of a large proportion of their power input. The signal response to the programming pattern usually picked up by their spiral DNA antenna falls weakened by a reduced power input from the blood. When the signal strengths from the organ cells falls, at the same time that there is a rapid change in the level of neuro-hormones from the thymus, then the suppresser activity of the t-lymphocyte cells can be reduced or fail completely. This allows the inducer t-lymphocyte to roar out of control unchecked. This can cause the white blood cells to attack the body's own native cells.

### POWER LOSS

In other words, robbed of their power supply by stress, the electronic activity in the cell diminishes. As this electronic activity diminishes, the cell transceiver which picks up and rebroadcasts the overall DNA instructions from the brain, powers down. As its signal reduces so does the strength of its protective field. If the immune system is hard at work removing a potential danger nearby, then the highly charged immune system cells can be stronger than the protective fields of the normal body cells and attack them. This is one of several high power state forms of cancer triggered by stress. Another of these is where a gene has been dislodged as follows.

### TRANSLOCATED GENES

A shock, neglect or abuse during the formative years, can cause hyper-irritation. If this is directed inwards it can dislodge a gene from its place on the chromosome. This gene then lodges in a different place on the chromosome. The chromosome is the basic spiral controller apparatus of every cell. This translocated gene in its original location was part of the control structure which was organising and directing the rapid growth of childhood. Rapid growth in infants and young people is achieved by rapid and controlled cell division. If a "rapid growth by division" gene is translocated to the wrong place on the control chromosome. There it stays surrounded by genes coded for more sophisticated instructions. Like a land mine waiting to explode when its triggered.

### SHOCK OR HYPER-IRRITATION

Later in life a physical injury or emotional blow can cause hyper-irritation. If this hyper-irritation is internalised it dumps hormones into the body. This is part of the stress related healing process. These hormones are the chemical messengers which cause rapid cell division, usually of normal light life cells. But if one of these translocated genes is lying buried in the early part of the chromosome. This can be triggered by hyper-irritation neuro-hormone levels which give it, as far as it's concerned, the wrong signals. It is coded for the rapid cell division growth process of early life but there are no "stop" instructions. Cancer is again often the result and this can happen in otherwise perfectly healthy seemingly unstressed people. It's the result of the tragic combination of early growth instructions with later healing instructions. This form of cancer is very difficult for the body's immune system to deal with because it operates behind a stronger defensive shield. However in time and given the right treatment the immune system can deal with this as with all other forms of cancer, provided it hasn't gone too far.

### THE COHERENT GENE

The question of power supply in the body is very important because when it drops or falls off, then the genes no longer have the energy to pick up and act on the body's "patterning" force. In each cell genes arranged in the complex spiral of the DNA are the code for life, life's pattern. But the pattern itself is no more than a form or a set of basic instructions with no activity. Only when you get activity do you see life emerge and function. So the genes themselves are not active instructions but more like musical instruments waiting for a player. In fact the genetic coding has sixty-four half tones which is about the same number as a cello and each of these half tones respond to a different specific UV wave length. One of the players of this orchestra is the chord of extremely low frequency resonances originating in the sun. This is one of the power suppliers of light life which shape and form all life on earth according to the make-up of each species genetic antenna.

### THE SEVEN TONES

In human beings the brain and spinal chord provide a superb antenna with seven areas of particular focus. These have traditionally been called the chakras. This antenna. picks up and focuses the major solar chord as well as components of the geomagnetic field. It then amplifies and rebroadcasts this in different proportions or notes of a coherent tone, throughout the body. This energy then causes the various gene antenna to oscillate with coherent frequencies at different levels of activity. These oscillations produce a consistent patterning of material. It is this patterning broadcast that brings order to the otherwise chaotic nature of growth. This pattern of rhythms which occur to a definite time sequence, throughout the body, are what caused the ordered formation of structures. From the single cell to the whole human body, these are the growth instructions of light life.

### ASYMMETRY

When a carbon atom is linked in a tetrahedral way to four different atoms, then two geometrically different molecules are formed. These are mirror images of each other. One molecule deflects a beam of light to the right and one to the left. Although they are made up of the same atoms, they have different electromagnetic structures because of the way they are assembled. All the amino acids in the body exist only in the left-handed form. Because an electric current can only produce a left-handed field. They are organised in this way by the complex of wave forms set up in the body by the action of the patterning force broadcast from the brain-spine antenna.

### THE ELECTRO-IMMUNE SYSTEM

This organising factor is particularly important in the understanding of cancer and the electro-immune system. If a cell is either deprived of adequate power to respond to its patterning signal, or if it is "shunted" out of its patterned structure, by shock or stresses of the kind we mentioned earlier, then, the immune system can attack it. This is possible because the now disorganised cell will rebalance to contain molecules of a right-handed nature. These have a different electromagnetic structure from the molecules organised by the life force. Substances with different electromagnetic properties have different chemical expressions — they taste, smell and behave differently and right-handed structures are basically non-organic and are consequently attacked by the defence agents of the left-handed life form. This bears directly on the subject of illness.

### SPINS

A molecule is held in balance by electrons spinning around the proton. In organic substances electrons spin in opposite directions in what is known as a singleton state. Magnetic fields interact with matter by influencing the movement of electrons. The movement of electrons from molecule to molecule can cause unstable states. These occur when electrons are pushed to spinning in parallel, the triplet state, before returning to their normal balance in the opposing spin singleton state. In these interactions highly unstable molecules can spin off and these scavenge for electrons with which to pair. These are called free radicals and are quite dangerous in some circumstances.

### THE HYPERFINE INTERACTION

Usually free radicals find an electron acceptor/electron with which to pair and become stable again. However, if too many of them are created by the electromagnetic field, then their field strength can be higher than the normal cohesive bonds holding the electrons in place in a molecule. When this happens they have enough power to overcome the local magnetic field of the molecule. They can then rob electrons from stable molecules, altering their electromagnetic make-up.

### SPIN REVERSAL

As we saw in asymmetry, molecules are made up of atoms. These atoms have electrons which spin in different directions. If a free radical steals an electron from one of these which has an opposing spin, then the entire chemical structure of that atom can change into the right-handed form. The non-life form. The immune system can normally deal with this situation. However, if this happens on a large enough scale it can overwhelm the ability of the immune system to respond. When this happens a minor change at the beginning of the reaction can become amplified further along the biological chain. This dramatically alters the chemical structure in that area of the body. It creates concentrations of right-handed chemical molecules — the mirror image non-life form. The result of this is the changed electronic potential — imbalance and ill-health.

## CHAPTER THREE

## *HEALTH POWER*

So far we've seen that cancer is actually an earlier life form that exists within all of us and we've seen what at base, causes cancer in terms of cellular power loss causing aberrant or inappropriate genetic signals. But there is something else we've seen and this is something demonstrated by millions of people all over the world every day:

THE BODY'S IMMUNE SYSTEM CAN HANDLE CANCER. YOUR OWN BODY, ESPECIALLY IF IT'S GIVEN A LITTLE HELP, CAN "CURE" YOU OF CANCER AND KEEP YOU FREE OF IT!

Daily throughout the world people with cancer experience spontaneous remission. Their body's cure themselves, they get better. This is a scientific and medical fact, so let's examine now how this happens.

### STRESS

The main control functions of the human body are provided by the nervous system and the glandular system. Broadly speaking nerves work on an electrical basis with signals being transmitted to the brain by a hard wired system of neuro-pathways. Once these signals reach the brain action is initiated in a number of ways, one of the most important of which is the stimulation of the glandular system. The glandular system controls the internal environment of the body via the bloodstream and lymph, and it does this by secreting different neuro-hormonal substances into the blood. These cause shifts in the balance of the body by amplifying or diminishing the activity in different areas as a response to the signals that the nerves have sent to the brain.

Activity is amplified or diminished by cells in the area being stimulated to higher or lower rates of activity by the neuro-hormones, they either damp down or become very active and often replicate strongly. In this way neuro-hormones act as the body's main stimulant to cellular activity, or put another way, as their main irritant. There are several other messenger and signalling systems within the body, since nature wisely never relies solely on one system, however this one serves to illustrate quite well that stress in one form or another is an integral part of the control system of life in the body. Stress causes cells to divide in order to be able to perform their function better and stress causes them to die when they are exhausted.

Stress mediates life and controls it but stress is not life, it simply helps to define its contours. Life is the interplay of many subtle forces having its physical aspect in this dimension but life in the electromagnetic sense is the flow of electrons through the body in response to demands set up by thousands of interrelated dynamic systems at work. None of these systems can live or perform work without this flow and it is to the optimisation of this flow which we should look to help ourselves when we get cancer (which we all do from time to time).

## WHERE POWER COMES FROM

The body derives power from air, food, water and light. It also derives power from the resonances in the cavity between the surface of the earth and the ionosphere (usually caused by thunderstorms). It gets power from the electronic activity of falling water in the form of fine rain. It gets power from the sympathetic resonances set up by harmonic sounds. It gets power from the earth's fluctuating electromagnetic field flowing through the meridians, it gets power from negatively charged winds and it gets power from love. All these and many other power sources are measurable scientific phenomena and they all contribute to the make-up of the power input into the human form.

In order to recharge an over-stressed cellular system it's important to understand how these various power input systems work within the human body so that you can consciously help them. You consciously help them by later learning to focus your mind and redirect your life, but for the moment let's look at how the spiral form of energy flow has been adapted over the millions of years of our evolution to act as a power source as well as the means of power transmission in living systems.

### VORTICES

If you take a hose pipe, anchor one end, and twist it, it will begin to curve. If you twist it further it will begin to curl up into a spiral. In this form it will not kink or collapse, and will always spring back into its original strong spiral form after it's been stressed in any way. Every structure in the body is made this way. It is the strongest structure in nature and the most dynamic.

### PULSATION

When you pass water down the spiral armature you can often see the whole thing throb or pulse in response to variations in the flow of the water. This pulsation too is a function of spirals that nature uses in life forms as we shall see, and this is where our journey into new understanding begins.

### THE SECOND LAW OF THERMO-DYNAMICS

According to this law, without further or continuous input of energy, all (closed) systems must degenerate into a condition of total chaos or entropy. In terms of passing fluid down or through a pipe this means that as the fluid flows along, friction is set up between the fluid and the sides of the pipe. This friction builds up and creates turbulence which cuts down the energy of the fluid flow. It takes energy out of the equation.

Now that normally holds good in ordinary situations where hydraulic engineers are using smooth bore pipes to transmit a fluid, but that "law" simply doesn't apply to living systems or to any system which copies nature.

### NATURE

All nature uses the spiral wound form to convey fluids and

energy, but in nature these spirals have one fundamental addition to their structure. They all contain an internal double rifled structure, they have internal spiral helixes. This adds a spin to everything going through the pipe in the same way that rifling in a gun spins a bullet, making it go farther and faster, (so too does nature add a spin to liquids and energy). The difference is that the barrel of a gun is straight so it only does half the job whereas the path of our arteries is laid out in a spiral and that spiral provides the missing element.

### SPIRAL HELICAL STRUCTURES

Spiral helical structures like all those used in nature to convey fluids do not set up friction in the course of performing work, rather they add energy!

When fluid passes down a tube which is set in a spiral form and has an internal double helix then it can pass through this in a frictionless state. The degree of friction or conversely of negative friction (= energy input) is governed by the velocity or pressure at which the fluid is presented to the tube. At an optimum pressure, which is governed by the volume of the tube, the number of turns in the helix, and the temperature of the fluid, the fluid can derive energy from the action of the vortices set up by its movement down the tube. Further if the tube is subjected to rhythmic pulses, these can cause yet more slippage and pressure differentials to be set up in the fluid which increase its dynamism and available energy.

### THE ENERGY SPIRAL

To understand how energy is derived from a rifled spiral tube it is as well to look at how energy flows through a spiral vortex and what happens to it as a resultant force in the form of suction. In a whirlpool the movement of the outer rim is quite slow. But as the lines of force begin to fold over each other and pull the centre into a striated cone, the forces become very much stronger. These set up a resultant force which is generally at right angles to the movement of the hole. This force passes from the lower pressure at the top of the vortex down through the higher pressure below the surface of the fluid. It consolidates and accelerates the lines of force as it revolves inwards forming an even stronger convergent force as it does so. This action continually reduces friction on the external plane of the cone (the tube walls) by pulling fluid away from the walls. It also continually adds power to the generally right-angular force of suction in the centre. This is how all naturally occurring forces move — they don't throw power out — they suck it in and increase its usefulness.

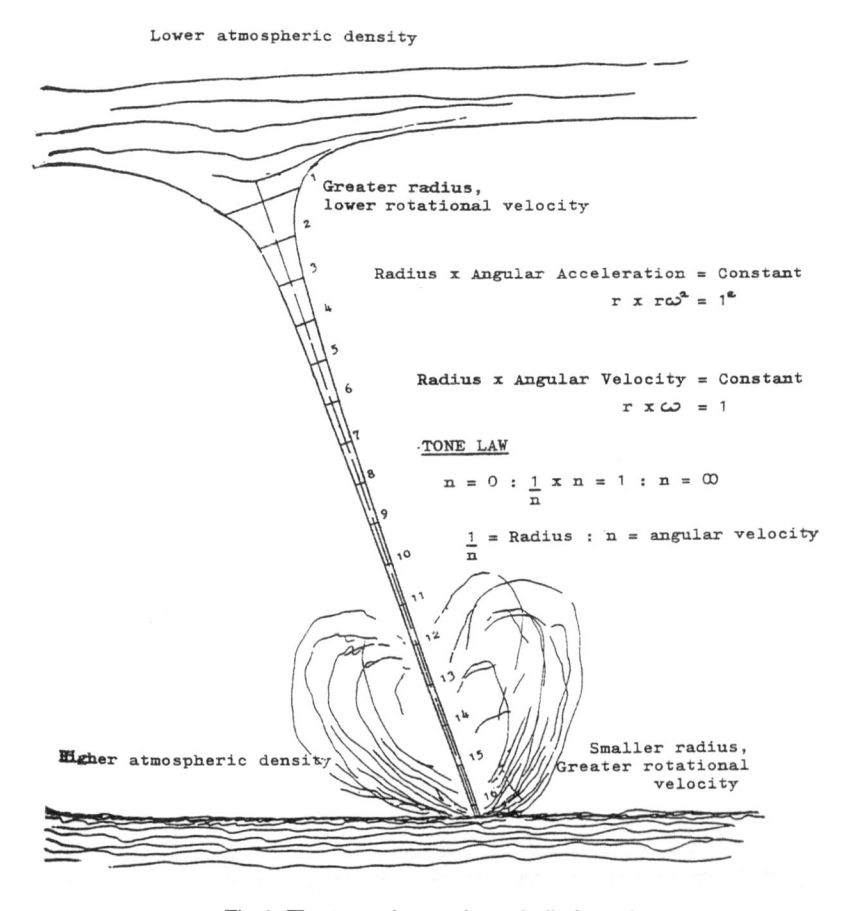

Lower atmospheric density

Greater radius, lower rotational velocity

Radius x Angular Acceleration = Constant
$r \times r\omega^2 = 1^2$

Radius x Angular Velocity = Constant
$r \times \omega = 1$

TONE LAW

$n = 0 : \frac{1}{n} \times n = 1 : n = \infty$

$\frac{1}{n}$ = Radius : $n$ = angular velocity

Higher atmospheric density

Smaller radius, Greater rotational velocity

Fig 1  The tornado as a hyperbolic funnel

## CENTRIPETAL FORCE

The winding-in force or centripetal force is the only way that a large low energy system can be transmuted into a concentrated high energy system. It also provides the best method of compressing and transmitting matter through narrow tubes. In the human body the life forces take all the slight and gentle forces of nature and twists them into a concentrated force of great strength using the inward flowing concentrating force of the vortex spiral as their mechanism.

## BLOOD CIRCULATION

In this way blood is sucked around the body by the arteries rather than being pumped around by the heart. (Incidentally the heart is far too small to be able to pump blood round the body, it would need a much bigger stronger organ to do the job, the heart is actually a pulsing device evolved to give the energy kick needed to pulsate the system.)

## CELLULAR RECHARGE

Health anomalies of any kind in the human body all depend on healthy cellular activity. This healthy cellular activity depends entirely on cellular respiration, and healthy cellular respiration depends on a steady and regular supply of electrons to the cells. The way that the bloodstream supplies electrons is via the arterial blood. Basically the bloodstream consists of two interconnected systems - the arteries and the veins. The arteries whirl the blood out to the farthest reaches of the body and the veins bring it back assisted by a series of non-return valves evolved to help with its increased viscosity and low electronic activity.

Arterial blood picks up oxygen from the lungs. This oxygen has a net negative charge and so the bright red oxygen-rich arterial blood takes on a negative charge which means it's rich in electrons and very active. It distributes this blood throughout the body via the millions of arterial capillaries which bring it into direct contact with the cells. As mentioned earlier no cell in the human body is more than a couple of cells away from the capillary. Blood is made up of blood cells and serum and where the space is too small at the wall of a capillary to allow a blood cell through, then serum is squirted through to nourish the cells and clean the debris away. This later returns to the blood stream as lymph.

Cells use the electrons from oxygen and give out carbon as a waste product. This bonds to the electron-depleted oxygen to become carbon dioxide and this carbon dioxide is dissolved into the venous blood. Because the carbon in this equation has a positive charge, the blood in the veins has a net positive charge. (The positive and negative aspects of the blood flow were first recorded by Bjorn E.W Nordenstroom M.D., Professor of Diagnostic Radiology at the Karolinska Institutet Stockholm, Sweden in his book "Biologically Closed Electric Circuits"). The carbon dioxide in the positive stream is dispelled through the lungs as we breathe out and the whole cycle begins again.

### HEART BEAT

There is however another important function that the negatively charged arterial blood and the positively charged venous blood perform whilst in this system — they trigger the heart beat!

Since these two types of blood carry opposite charges, the muscular contraction and closing action of the heart is triggered through the periodic equalisation of positive and negative charges, which reach a maximum in the venal and arterial chambers of the heart itself, due to the large charge carrying volume of both.

The heart isn't really a pump at all. It's actually a device that nature has evolved to promote a pulsation in the flow of blood. This pulsation is driven by us breathing in negatively charged oxygen and breathing out positively charged carbon dioxide (and water). The purpose of the pulsation is to drive the system of arteries. Each pump/throb of the heart causes a spasm in the blood vessels which draws the frictionless flow of blood through the complex of capillaries which supply the cellular cooperatives in the body. As blood is sucked round this system its velocity/speed is dictated by the optimum flow configuration of each tube as it expands and contracts to the pulses coming via the resonant cavities in the body to each tube wall. The viscosity of the blood decreases in inverse proportion to the diameter of the blood vessels owing to the range of pressure derived from the pulsations. And this fall in viscosity in the capillaries is a direct result of the way in which the blood is torqued as it passes through the system.

The body acts like a giant sponge sucking the blood and lymph into and out of its tissues.

### BACTERIA, HEAT AND $CO_2$

When blood is drawn along a spiral vessel which has three or more parallel systems of guide vanes inside it the fluid takes on flow characteristics which allow it to adjust its viscosity to suit the branching of smaller or larger capillaries. It also cleans and disinfects itself in the process. This is the mechanism:

The section or characteristics of the blood vessel set up longitudinal vortexes. These are not simple vortices but double spiral ones. The central main blood flow describes a single spiral motion while the peripheral flow describes a double motion. (It rotates around itself, while at the same time spiralling around the central core like a smoke ring). The outer ring of blood by roiling round on itself, acts as a sort of ball-bearing between the inner core blood and the blood vessel wall. It conveys oxygen and nutrients from the central core of the blood to the walls of the blood vessel and carries carbon waste products back. The stripping action of this helically toroidal flow draws pathogenic bacteria from the vessel walls when they are then attacked and overwhelmed by the aggressively oxygenated blood of the central core and eliminated.

This physical process is aided and abetted by an electronic process whereby negatively charged oxygen is attracted to bacteria which have a net positive charge. It shorts them out! (It should be noted here that bacteria use the fermentation process to provide themselves with energy and are therefore more electro-positive than the negatively charged arterial oxygen).

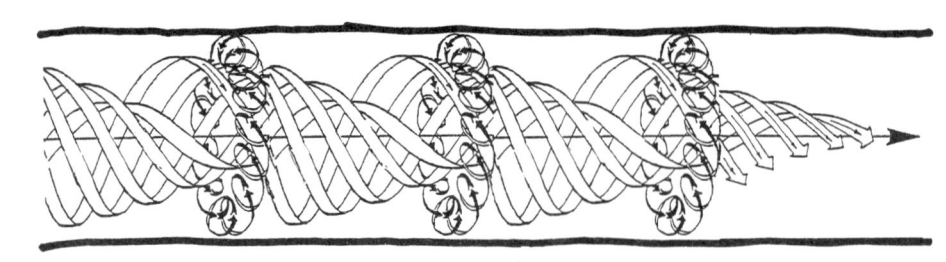

Fig 2  A Helically Toroidal Flow

Because of the build up of carbon waste products in the course of cellular respiration/function, the walls of the blood vessels are sites of a more electro-positive charge than the highly oxygenated and therefore more negatively charged blood flowing through them. This causes the two charges to be attracted to one another when the resultant detoxified debris is stripped away into the bloodstream.

Heat is also transferred from the vessel walls (tissue) to the blood by the action of the "roller bearing" outer blood vortex and this serves to redistribute and regulate the overall body temperature.

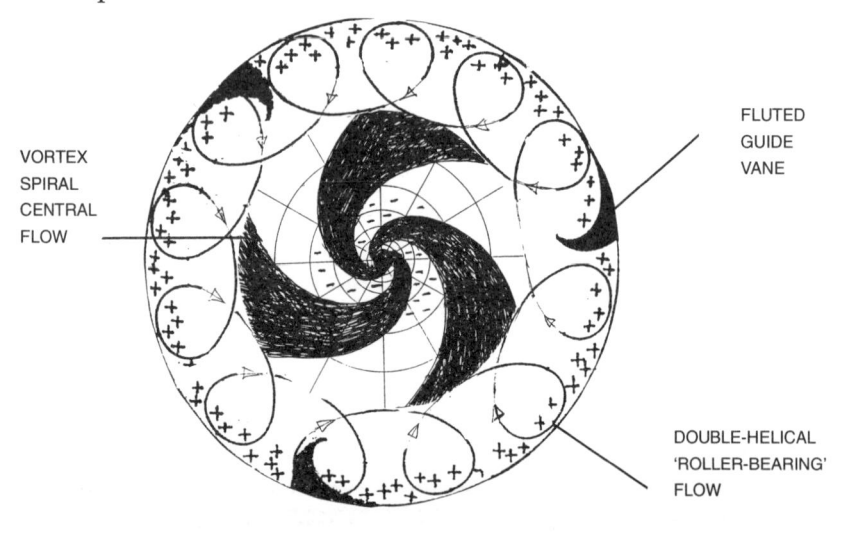

Fig 3  The 'Roller Bearing' Vortex

The presence of the outer roller bearing vortex allows for a frictionless flow of blood through the central core. Since this is continually acted on by the pull of its own vortex form it exerts a strong suction along its length which transports oxygen (and electrons) to the further reaches of the body.

SUMMARY

To summarise then the system of tubes developed by nature to convey blood around the body has several well known characteristics. It's all part of an inter-twining and inter-connecting two-tree system of spirals. These spirals all have striations or double helixes the characteristic of their cross section, and these spiral helixes are capable of sucking the blood around the body in a frictionless supply.

Because of the negative and positive charges set up in the blood by the function of cellular respiration, the heart complex of organs spasms rhythmically to equalise these charges. This sets up a pressure peak in the spiral system causing them to throb or pulse, and this pulse flows throughout the system in the form of a wave of energy which alters the section of the blood-carrying vessel and thus sucks the blood around the system. It does this by flexing/energising the system along its entire length with each percussion and thus establishes the rhythmic pulsation of life.

The blood being drawn through this system divides into a central core which is subject to a high degree of suction by its passage through the vessels. This central core acts as the main transport agent of the blood supply carrying an initially high proportion of dissolved oxygen. The secondary component of the blood flow is the section initially "spun" by the outer vessel walls. This component roils along the walls acting as a bearing for the central core, whilst at the same time conveying oxygen to the vessel walls from the central flow and carrying bacteria and carbon dioxide from the walls into the central flow. In the process this roiling flow functions as a very active bactericide and heat transfer mechanism, cleaning and cooling the body tissues it passes through. It also conveys a vital supply of electrons throughout the body. These electrons are the basis of healthy cellular function and are drawn from the ocean of air in which we live.

### ACTIVE AIR

Air is not usually thought to be a good conductor of electricity but without the movement of electrons in the air no life, as we know it could exist on earth. In the same way as all other matter, air is made up of molecules. In the case of air these molecules are of gas and of water vapour. Each molecule has a core of positively charged protons surrounded by outer shells of negatively charged electrons. In a passive or stable molecule of air these charges cancel each other out. however in the healthy normal conditions which apply outdoors in a forested living environment, the air is rarely stable.

An electron is 1,800 times lighter than a proton and is quite easily displaced. When that happens the equilibrium between the positive and the negative charges is upset and an unstable molecule or ion is created.

The ability of an electric charge (a flow of electrons) to pass through the air, depends on these ions, and as we have seen all life depends on electron flow. The more dynamic the flow the more vital the life force!

> The flow mechanism is as follows:
> If a molecule loses an electron it becomes more positively charged (because it has just lost a little bit of its negative charge), conversely if a displaced electron attaches itself to a normal molecule then that molecule becomes negatively charged, (it's just gained an extra bit of negative power).
> 
> The energy needed to displace electrons comes from minute radio-active sources in the soil, from the lightning in thunderstorms, of which there are about 2,000 going on in the earth's atmosphere at any one time, from fine droplets of water falling through the air near waterfalls, fountains or in light rain showers, from the action of the earth's geomagnetic field along the surface of the globe, and increasingly these days, from the dangerous levels of radiation emitted by radar and microwave transmitters.

## INTENTIONAL IONS

They can also be generated artificially using an avalanche circuit originally invented by Sir John Cockroft, later developed and improved by the brilliant "Coppy" Laws and finally engineered to perfection by the practical genius Derek Smith. This device is known as a "Progenitor".

Ions come in three sizes, large clusters, medium size positive ions and small size negative ions. It's the small negative ions which are used by plants and human tissue to support cellular respiration, simply because it's easier to part the spare electron from a negative ion and pass this on to be used in cellular function.

In fresh air over open countryside there are between one and two thousand ions in every cubic centimetre of air. The usual ratio is five positive to four negative and it's generally in this ion balance and ratio that life evolved. Air ions are essential to life and the more negative ions that are available in a given body of air then the more active the flow of electrons.

## PLANT GROWTH

In one experiment on ionisation scientists at the University of California grew barley, oats, lettuce and peas with a total of only sixty positive and negative ions. They found that growth was stunted and the plants became rapidly diseased in this atmosphere. The same experiment was conducted in air with more than double the natural number of ions and this produced accelerated and healthy growth!

In Russia D.A. Lapitsky used a similar experiment on small animals showing their sensitivity to ion levels. He placed animals in an atmosphere depleted of oxygen, and as they were about to die of suffocation, he added negative ions and found that animals already near death from asphyxiation began to feel better. They sat up sniffed the air and began to run around the chamber. Their respiration frequency increased and they became healthy despite the low oxygen level!

Switching off the ioniser again brought them to the verge of asphyxiation and it was concluded that death of animals in filtered (de-ionised) air must be attributed to the absence of aero-ions of oxygen essential to the life activity of an organism.

### AIR CONDUCTIVITY

Basically it's all a question of the conductivity which exists between a living organism and its surrounding environment. Where there is a normal balanced proportion of ions in the surrounding atmosphere, a body can interact with the surrounding atmosphere taking in and giving out the continual flow of positive and negative ions needed to pump its metabolic systems.

Where the conductivity of the air is high — in the presence of a high negative ion count, then the electron flow in the human body takes on a very considerably higher vitality. This vitality acting as a stimulus or pump to cellular activity, accelerates growth, healing and restructuring by enabling a greater degree of electronic activity to take place in the proteins (the basic building blocks of life).

As we have seen earlier negatively charged oxygen also acts as a strong bactericide and viricide since it combines very strongly with the net positive charges generated by the life functions of these entities, knocking them into a state of suspended animation.

This counterflow of energy to and from the air has a vital function in living systems and is yet another power source used by the life force.

### POWER LEACHING AIR

Air in buildings contains little or no ionic charge as all its electronic activity is shorted-out onto the positively charged surfaces of the buildings interior and its contents. This positive charge derives from friction and in fact those buildings having air-conditioning and central heating systems suffer worst since virtually every biologically available negative charge is stripped out of their air as it is drawn in through the metal grills and conduits of the air-conditioning system. These conduits pick up a strong positive charge from the friction of the air flow and this charge "denatures" the air of its healthy electron content very rapidly.

This is why illness spreads so quickly through air-conditioned buildings and why listlessness, lethargy and headaches develop so quickly as precursors of Sick Building Syndrome.

As we saw from the earlier experiments any environment low in, or devoid of, a balance of charges in the air is inimical to life since it is capable of stripping electrons from the body. As we shall see later in this chapter this can be a contributory factor in the onset of cancer, which is caused at base by a lack of electrons in dividing cells.

## WITCH WINDS

There are circumstances in the natural outdoor world where the air can be harmful to living systems. These occur in areas of the world where a wind blows continually over a dry land mass. The friction set up by its passage and the fact that it picks up no water drops, means that it develops a positive charge. This positive charge is capable of drawing the opposing negative charges out of any organic or living system it comes into contact with, and, in the case of mammalian systems, when it leaches out some of their negative charge they become prone to illness and disease. (The same as the animals in Lapitsky's experiments).

The Santa Anna in California, the Sharav in Israel, the Hamma Tan in Arabia, The Mistral in France, the Fhn in the Alps, the Scirocco, and a whole range of similar devil/witch winds are examples of this phenomenon. They raise the levels of the neuro-hormone seratonin in the blood, make people as irritable as hell and cause very destructive behaviour. On a miniature scale this is what happens to living systems trapped in buildings with no healthy balanced air flow — the electronic gradient between the living system and the atmosphere, favours the outflow of electrons and the living system "flags" accordingly.

## THUNDER STORMS, LIGHTNING AND RAIN

Similarly, the oppressive feeling experienced before a thunder storm is caused by the build-up of excessive positive charge in the air/clouds above the earth, which is "shorted out" and released by flashes of lightning.

Lightning occurs when the polarised potentiality between the atmospheric positive charge and the earth's negative charge become so great as to overcome the natural reluctance of the air to conduct a large electrical charge.

To flow as lightning the charge has to polarise/ionize vast amounts of air, and this imbalance in airborne charges is the active component in the resultant rain. Rain makes these minute parcels of energy available to living systems.

## SPIRAL BREATHING

Because electrons are quite easily stripped from negative ions, especially when they come into contact with the tissues of the body, mammals have developed a method of preserving these in the air whilst it is being transported to the lungs.

As with the bloodstream the mechanism is the spiral helical armature. Air is drawn into the body mainly through the nose. The inner surfaces of the nose have a spiral form the same as all other structures in the body. Into this spiralling airflow there intrude first a dense mass of hairs pointing generally outward (i.e. against the inward airflow), these hairs act as vanes which impart a toroidal spin to the outer area of the airflow (remember the roller bearing effect in the bloodstream) and this separates the inner air flow from the walls of the nasal passage thus allowing/helping it maintain and transport an electronically active supply of fresh air to the lungs. If this were not the case all the charges held in the airflow would short out onto the sides of the nose in the first couple of centimetres of their passage into the body.

Later in the bronchial passages this spinning function is taken on by the cillia and these small whip-like appendages are actually stimulated into frenzied activity by the presence of a high level of negative charge in the air.

Once again this is a function of velocity and the cillia whip to maintain the vortex flow so that the maximum amount of negatively charged oxygen can reach the lungs and be absorbed by the blood. (The cillia also remove debris and bacteria from the air stream, passing these back up into the nose and throat to be expelled as phlegm).

All the body's systems co-operate very strongly to supply the component cells with the healthy active wherewithal to support life, and cooperation not competition, is the hallmark of healthy living systems.

CHAPTER FOUR

*THE LATTICE OF LIFE*

The earth is in the outer atmosphere of the sun where it is subjected to a continual bombardment of electromagnetic radiation. This bombardment is known as the photon wind or solar wind. It is made up mostly of light in the visible spectrum and infra-red radiation with a small component of just under 1 per cent of ultra-violet. The sun vibrates like a vast jelly at rhythms of every five minutes to rhythms of just over 1 hour. These vibrations are caused by the huge nuclear reaction in the sun's core. This thunders away hurling vast quantities of energy (mainly electrons and protons) which fling away from the sun into space.

THE MAGNETOSPHERE

The solar wind compresses the earths magnetic field on the sunward side to within eight to ten earth radii. On the other side it draws it out into a long magnetotail like a ship's wake. The earth spirals around the sun whilst the solar wind blows past it. This means that the magnetosphere is moving through the magnetic field of the sun at a speed about eight times faster than the speed of sound.

BOW WAVE

This acts to build up a bow wave or bow shock between the earth and the solar wind. This bow wave in the magnetosphere forms a shell or protective layer around the earth. It exists about three to four earth radii out from the sunward side. Because this layer is compressed by the action of the solar wind, the constant changes in the solar wind output make it vibrate. As we've seen earlier the sun is continually vibrating and these vibrations impact on the protective layer of the bow shock around the earth.

## SEVEN DRUMS

Between the bow wave of the magnetosphere and the surface of the earth there are seven layers of protection. The first of these is the Van Allen belts which occupy two zones at about 1.5 and 5 earth radii respectively. These contain charged particles which spiral between the north and south pole trapped by the earth's magnetic field. In the far north you can sometimes see these as the aurora borealis (the northern lights) and in the south as the aurora australis (the southern lights). The next layer of protection is the ionosphere and there are four regions of ionisation in the upper atmosphere. The closest is the d region extending up to 90 kilometres above ground level where it reflects long wave lengths of radiation. Variations in the ionosphere caused by solar activity influence the frequence and intensity of thunderstorms on the earth's surface. In this way solar activity drives the earth's weather.

The final layer of protection for life on earth is the ozone layer which exists about 20 to 30 kilometres above the earth's surface. This absorbs ultraviolet radiation.

## THE CHORD

Each of the protective belts around the earth acts as a shield or buffer, preventing different forms of radiation from impacting on the earth's surface. Each of these buffers is constantly battered by variations in the level of radiation coming from the sun. Each buffeting transmits shock waves through the resonant cavity formed between the shield and the surface of the earth. Each of these balloon like cavities have different characteristics of resonance. They are all different shapes and sizes. They all vibrate at different frequencies in different keys. Each one handles a different form of (long wave, ultraviolet, x-rays and etc.) energy and they all pass on different levels of energy to earth. This is the fluctuating and vibrating background chord of extremely low frequency sound energy, against which life has evolved since light first reached the surface of our planet.

## PATTERNS OF RHYTHMIC ACTIVITY

Living systems were first clumped together into co-operating structures by the very low frequency sound waves of thunder. From the very beginning life on earth has used every single available energy source to its purpose and benefit. The life force has never abandoned any energy source but simply learnt to use it more effectively to build up more complex structures. The spiralling extremely low frequency energy provided by the sun's wind buffeting the earth's shield is no exception. It is used by all life to build patterns out of matter. Its coherence or repeating rhythms are essential to life and health. It provides the major component in the patterning force which organises and keeps on organising living systems in dynamic cooperatives. It is part of the lattice of life.

The moon adds a further component to this lattice by pumping the ionosphere as follows:

### THE FLOW

The ionosphere blocks out some of the flow of charged particles flung out from the sun. These flow around it like water round a ball. This flow gives it an electrical charge. This charge effectively polarises the ionosphere so that the top which faces outer space is negatively charged, and the under side that faces the earth is positively charged. The interaction between the positively charged underside and the negatively charged earth is a key element in the generation and activity of ions in the air. The moon is the mechanism that drives their flow.

### THE MOON

The moon orbits the earth outside the ionosphere. It is negatively charged like the earth. When the moon is full it's closer to the earth than at any other time. Its charge repels the negative outer face of the ionosphere pushing it closer to the earth. This causes a stronger interaction between the positively charged underside of the ionosphere and negatively charged earth. The number of positive ions drawn down to the surface increases and the number of negative ions repelled by the surface increases. A stronger flow is established. This flow spirals up and down the left and right-handed magnetic lines of force created between the magnetosphere and the geomagnetic field. The negative ions follow the left-handed spirals. This "handedness" of air electricity is very important to a further understanding of cancer as we saw in the spin reversal section at the end of Chapter Two.

### THE LUNAR PUMP

Effectively, the moon's monthly cycle pumps the ionosphere up and down. This pumping action affects all life on earth because it modulates the electronic activity which can take place in cellular structures. As the moon waxes more ions flow. As they flow, more electrons fizz between them. The air becomes more highly energised. Human life utilises this energy in two ways. Firstly the blood supply becomes more negatively charged. It is able to absorb more electrons from the air in the lungs. It becomes more vital. Secondly, these air borne electrical charges pass straight through specific areas of the skin to charge various "cooperatives".

### THE PATHWAYS

No clear boundary exists between the bodies metabolically maintained electromagnetic fields and those of its environment. There are over 1,000 locations on the human body at the skin's surface which have a much lower electrical resistance than the rest of the skin. These are often referred to as acupuncture points and are small areas usually invisible to the naked eye. These points all connect up to a series of electron "pathways" in the body. There are fourteen main pathways and several subsidiaries. Each of the pathways passes through a series of related organs and they all conduct the diurnal flow of electrons.

## THE DOUBLE HELIX CONTRA-FLOW OF POWER

Electrons from the air and the earth, when flowing up and down through living systems, not only provide sources of extra cellular energy, but they also provide an essential patterning element to the flow of life. Without this there would be no growth blue print. Simply put, at the points where they intersect, these force matrixes contribute the energy nexus which react with the patterning signals from the DNA of the living system, to provide the interference pattern or hologram which dictates the form which the life force should follow. These opposing force flows form the yin and yang of Taoist philosophy and are the bedrock of one of the most effective and sophisticated systems of medicine in use in the world. Here is how these flows are formed:

> The earth has a hot core of liquid molton rock which is subjected to movement because of the planet's spin. This spin takes place within the earth's magnetic field and sets up a generator effect causing the earth to have many of the properties of a giant electro-magnet. Lines of electromagnetic force issue from the core which ripples as it dissipates the energy caused by the spin. These waves of energy reach the surface of the earth in a steadily pumped flow of extremely low frequency electromagnetic energy. This, like the earth it comes from, has a negative charge. At the surface of the earth it meets and reacts with the incoming extremely low frequency electromagnetic energy from the sun, planets and constellations. This incoming energy has a positive charge and flows across the surface of the planet like water across a ball. The two energy flows polarise into twin currents dependent upon one another, in all living systems. They serve to potentiate organic structures, that is to say they boost their electronic activity and energetic functions to a higher frequency.

The energy flowing from the earth has a net negative charge, the earth being electro-negative. Whereas the energy flowing from the sun has a net positive charge, the sun being a source of positive charges in space. These charges spiral together at the earth's surface to form interlocking double helixes and this is the form or energy flow that our early protein ancestors followed in forming the first steps on the DNA, the "pattern of life".

They are still at work in every organic structure on earth today and later we'll see how these can be strengthened or reinforced to help prevent illness.

## ACUPUNCTURE

As I mentioned earlier, the Chinese system of medicine is derived from Taoism, it suggests that health is achieved and disease prevented by maintaining the body in a balanced state. This system of Chinese belief states that two opposing forces exist in a natural world, yin and yang whose vital energy or "qi" circulates through the body and keeps these forces in balance. A normal fluctuating balance of yin and yang should exist in the healthy individual and the degree of fluctuation is what makes us feel better on some days than on others. Traditional Chinese medicine also contains a code of laws which govern the selection of acupuncture points and describe in exact detail the function of a whole variety of organs. In fact some of the organ functions described by the ancient Chinese, predate by many hundreds of years their discovery in the west. For instance the Chinese discovered the double circulation of blood long before western medicine realised that it existed.

## MERIDIANS

There are 14 main meridians connecting up the acupuncture points, eight of which are used largely for treating internal diseases and six of which are used in painful conditions. There are over 1,000 locations on the body at the skin's surface called acupuncture points, and although these are not distinguishable by any observable structural feature in the body tissue, the electrical resistance in the skin shows a decrease within a few millimetres of these points. Each relates to a specific and remotely situated body organ or function, which can be affected by some treatment at the appropriate acupuncture point.

In fact each of these meridians represents a macro-metabolic pathway conducting the flow of electrons through the body. During this flow they pass through a number of separate circulatory systems where their path follows the optimum course of conductivity. This flow of electrons or qi (pronounced key) can be interrupted if an organ it passes through is not functioning properly. This is another way of saying if an organ has an altered conductivity through some malfunction then the electrons don't flow smoothly through it but encounter resistance. The objective of most Chinese acupuncture in practice, is to correct the flow of qi through the body so as to bring malfunctioning organs back into their healthy optimum range of activity.

Acupuncture is accompanied by a philosophy of life that involves checks and balance which determine health or disease, and an understanding of how individuals can be made more healthy by being placed in electronically enriched environments where more negative charges are present. In acupuncture the life forces, body energy or qi, are supposed to circulate through the meridians day and night 25 times in each. This is another circadian rhythm in the body which is now scientifically provable.

### RADIOACTIVE PHOTOGRAPHY

Recent work by two doctors from Paris (Jean Claude Darras and Dr De Vernejoul) to test the validity of energy transport along the meridians, has succeeded in visualising these. A radio active trace (solutions containing one of the radio active isotopes; technetium, mercury or xenon) was injected at an acupuncture point and it was found, using a gamma-ray camera, that the radioactivity travelled along the acupuncture meridian at a velocity of three to five centimetres a minute. This is the right order of magnitude to give 25 circulations per day or night. It was also found that the circulation rate was slower in the case of diseased organs.

Also it was confirmed that the radioisotope did not diffuse

appreciably if injected other than at an acupuncture point. It did not enter into the lymphatic system or blood circulation but it did penetrate tourniquet preventing circulation. It only diffused towards the target organ if it was injected at an acupuncture point part way along the meridian, and the diffusion was not due to electro-phoretic forces because a non-ionic radio tracer (xenon) was equally affected.

The rate of diffusion along the meridian was increased when the acupuncture point was stimulated, whether by a needle or electrically by a helium neon laser. So now we can visualise this electron flow in the body.

Modern research is discovering many more acupuncture points covering the body, and these are all receptor areas for electrons passing through the skin in a continual flow to and from the surrounding electromagnetic environment.

Ions flowing through the atmosphere from the ionosphere to the earth and vice-versa, do so in tight spirals following the electromagnetically rotating field between the magnetosphere and the geomagnetic field. As these ions enter or exit the acupuncture sights on the skin of living organisms, they do so with a dextro (right-handed) or laevo (left-handed) rotation so that there is an electromagnetically rotating field which maintains a pressure in the direction of the organs served by that meridian.

The clouds of electrons in these fields can be captured on a photographic plate using an electron microscope where they have a distinct vortex form. The contours of each of these tiny rotating fields have exactly the same proportions as the main body chakras, and are formed at birth by the action of a complex of extremely low frequency electromagnetic force acting on the enzyme substrate of the DNA. In other words the entire bodily antenna is energised to the same pattern and degree at the moment it's "switched on". These different patterns in time affect the characteristic of all living systems, but for the moment suffice to say that electronic activity in each organ along this metabolic pathway is a contributory factor in the neuro-hormonal activity which takes place and which mediates the health of that organ and its contribution to the whole.

## CHAPTER FIVE

## *WATER ENERGY*

In a similar way to air, water isn't usually thought of as a bearer of energy or information, it's usually thought of simply as a basic compound of hydrogen and oxygen — simple $H_2O$.

In reality nothing could be further from the truth! Water is the original "living" substance on this planet. Under a microscope it continually flexes in response to the fluctuating electromagnetic field we've discussed earlier, passing through it. Whilst it's flexing and moving some areas in a body of water temporarily take on crystalline structures of ice before changing back into the polymer form of liquid water, at the same time other areas in the same body of water behave as though they are on the point of boiling.

Water is an amazing substance regarded by the great natural scientist and philosopher Victor Schauberger, as being not only the life blood of this planet and all things that live on it, but as having a character and function which made it the carrier of the life force.

### CLATHRATE SUBSTANCES

In theory water is composed of two atoms of hydrogen and one of oxygen. The formula $H_2O$ is therefore taken to represent the numbers of atoms in a molecule and the molecule of water is considered to be the smallest particle of water that can retain water's properties, (that can still be water). The atoms are thought to be the component parts of the molecule whose structural form is usually shown with a largish negatively charged oxygen atom (with two negative signs beside it) supported by two hydrogen atoms (which are smaller in size) each of which has a positive charge sign beside it.

This picture of the molecule structure presents a problem in relation to the subtle properties of water because water, even in its pure state, is capable of altering biological processes.

This means that pure water is able to accommodate information within its structure that is relevant to biological processes and the molecule model described above is not able to accommodate this fact.

In fact there is another dimension in the structure of water that accounts for its ability to affect biological processes. Water molecules are able to join together and form three-dimensional structures comprising a number of molecules. These form in such a way as to create a cage or shell with a space inside, technically known as a clathrate. These clathrates are known as the micro-structures of water and under certain conditions it's possible for other molecules to be trapped inside the cage of the micro-structures.

If you go back to the beginning of chapter one in the section "God's Voice Upon The Waters" you'll see where I allude to this capability of water when describing how water was shaken causing proteins to clump into organic patterns. This shaking or rhythmic vibration is one of the ways that water can be made to take in molecules of other substances and it's this unique capability of water that gave life its first foothold on the long ladder of evolution.

### MICRO-STRUCTURES

The micro-structures in water enable it to dissolve a very large range of substances, more than any other liquid. Many minerals, in fact most minerals, are slightly soluble in water, as are many gasses. (Unfortunately so are most of the 100,000 or so new, man-made substances that have found their way into the surface waters of the planet in the last century). These and other functions in water represent a major health hazard, as we shall see, and this whole capability of water to dissolve components of practically anything it comes in contact with plays a crucial role in what it transfers into the human body — in human health.

### ELECTROLYSIS

Described simply as $H_2O$ water is a dipole-molecule comprising two hydrogen atoms, one positive and one negative, and one negative oxygen atom containing two positive charges. Because of this structure pure distilled water has a dielectric value of 81. This means that it has a very high capacity to resist the transfer of an electric charge. In other words it's an extremely good insulator.

Since it's a good insulator, the idea that electrolysis can split it into two components is clearly an over-simplification since the current simply would not pass between the two plates (anode and cathode) which would be insulated by the water. Accordingly what's really happening in electrolysis is that the myriad impurities that water carries are conducting the charge and are what is precipitated out.

This is of paramount importance in looking at water's relationship to the human body, because not only does the body work on an electrical level, where differences of conductivity are all important, but it also works on a gross chemical level, where the ability of water to dissolve most things is crucial to its usefulness to the body.

Simply put then, without substances dissolved in it, water will not conduct an electric charge. Many of the functions of life are reliant upon and exemplified by a flow of electrons (an electric current). Therefore in order to be able to perform a function in living systems water must contain other substances in its micro-structures and the proportions of these substances will give to each body or quantity of water a specific/unique electromagnetic signature. Water with different subtle properties will have varying effects on the conductivity/activity of the body. So that water is very much more than a simple refreshing liquid but actually makes a contribution or otherwise to electronic activity in the body.

PROPERTIES

Basically water should be viewed in four ways:
1. It is a solvent.
2. As such it can take on a range of electro-chemical properties depending on what's dissolved in it.

3. These are affected by its temperature (which mediates its ability to dissolve more or less of a substance).
4. It has a high specific heat and thermal conductivity. (So that a large input or extraction of heat energy is required to bring about a change in its density and temperature).

This is very important to life because our blood is made up of up to 90 per cent water (or put another way our blood is water with 10 per cent of "impurities" added in). We each contain about 45 litres of water and consume about 2.4 litres a day. This consumption is used in every metabolic process in our bodies and without an input of water we die very quickly — usually within three days.

Viewed as a solvent water dissolves chemical complexes within us and transports these out of our bodies. However, water, because of its range of "dissolving" abilities will go on dissolving anything it comes into contact with until it reaches saturation at a particular temperature or density. Accordingly if the water we drink lacks some element, mineral or gas when it enters the body, it is capable of extracting this from the body as it passes through. In this way water can leach nutrients and chemicals from the body, just as easily as it can add them in. This is why if you try and live on distilled water you very soon become ill as the water is aggressively dissolving all the elements it needs out of your body.

ENERGY

Water is most dense and energetic at plus 4 degrees Celsius which is what is called its anomaly point. Whereas all other liquids become denser as they cool, water reaches its denser state at plus 4 degrees Celsius. Above or below this temperature it begins to expand and become lighter.

In relation to its anomaly point at plus 4 degrees Celsius water has two temperature gradients. A movement of temperature towards plus 4 degrees Celsius is a positive temperature gradient, and a movement of temperature away from plus 4 degrees Celsius is a negative temperature gradient.

As it flows water acts completely differently according to which ever temperature gradient is in force.

With cooling the volume decreases and the density increases, whereas with heating the opposite is the case.

This is important to us because heat or anything else dissolved or suspended in water always flows or is transported toward cold. This is a very significant function in the human body where fatty and often very toxic substances are deposited in areas of relative cold on the body — as CELLULITE.

Also water in process of moving toward or away from its anomaly point can either deposit or leach out oxygen from the body's tissue. As it is expanding with heat it takes up oxygen and conversely as its contracting with cold it gives it up. As it absorbs oxygen water increases in volume very substantially and the most crucial factor affecting the health and energy of creatures taking in water is its temperature.

SPECIFIC-HEAT CURVE

The most important aspect of water's temperature properties to us is its specific-heat curve. The lowest point of this is plus 37.5 degrees Celsius which is only .5 degrees Celsius above the average temperature of human blood.

This means that both water and blood (made up of 90 per cent water) are able to resist rapid thermal changes. The effect of this is to enable us to survive a large range of temperature changes and yet still maintain our body temperature. Without this ability we couldn't live in cold climates or hot climates and would become rapidly unviable as a species. Furthermore, if our body didn't have the tendency to return to this "home" temperature, then our immune system wouldn't be able to repair us nearly as well as it does.

So to summarise thus far:

> Water has the ability to transport chemical complexes into the human body, or it can leach them out. Water has a wide range of electro-chemical capabilities depending on what's dissolved in it and can transport these throughout the body. Finally water can add in or leach out heat energy until its

temperature reaches plus 37.5 degrees Celsius which is .5 degrees Celsius above the average heat of human blood.

So far we've seen how water's ability to dissolve just about anything to some degree or other makes it into an almost universal solvent, capable of carrying the most outlandish chemical cocktails into our bodies (or out)! So now let's look at water's other vital property: its ability to carry information.

VIBRATIONS

We've seen how water molecules are able to join together and form three dimensional structures made up of a number of molecules. These form in such a way as to make up a sort of cage which is technically known as clathrate. These micro-structures can hold other materials inside their cages, and these micro-structures are an important key to understanding water's information role in living structures.

Everything in nature has a natural rate of vibration. Everything fizzes with its own energy and this "fizzing" has a pitch or frequency which depends on its degree and type of molecular activity. Its molecular resonance.

However there is a substantial difference between resonance as we know it in the mechanical world and resonance in the molecular world. If you strike a bell it will ring for about half a minute and then the sound will fade away. That's how things work in the mechanical world. In the molecular world however this doesn't happen. When vibrations are imparted to a molecular structure (when their bell is rung) these vibrations never fade away. They're stored forever in that molecular structure either until they're supplanted by a stronger or different vibration or until that structure ceases to exist.

Water clathrate structures are capable of vibrating as a complete entity and are capable of being imprinted with vibrations from different material they come into contact with. The problem here however is that these vibrations then become permanent and fixed in the water.

Moreover because of the way they're structured (their three dimensional form), water clathrates are able to resonate and maintain not just one but a whole orchestra of vibrations.

MEMORY

The ability of water clathrates to memorise the vibrations of other substances permanently is not limited to the time when the other substance is present. These memories can be shown to remain in the water long after any trace of the original imprinting substance is gone (and this fact is the basis of homeopathy).

Details of the work of Dr Benoviste and his colleagues in Paris which proves this function of water were shown in the BBC Two documentary "Heretic" on 6th February 1994 and further results were published in "Nature" magazine volume 333 page 816.

MOVEMENT AND SPACE

Movement caused by vibration can form complex patterns in space. For example if you draw a bow up and down the edge of a metal plate covered in dust you will see the dust organised into shapes according to the speed of your bowing. These are called Chladni shapes. Or if you watch the dust on a speaker or amplifier you will see it clump into coherent shapes with the vibrations when music's being played. These examples demonstrate in the mechanical world the transfer of vibration into form and this is how life was first structured into water clathrates by the vibrations which drew the primitive amino-acid structures together at the dawn of life at this planet (as we've seen in Chapter One). However this function took place largely on a molecular level and therefore never dies away. These vibrations are still going on all the time in and around us and are permanently fixed in the clathrate structures of water as remembered forms!

PROPORTIONS

Every chemical element or compound has its own unique

vibratory pattern whether it's dissolved in water or not. A spectro-scope which passes light through a substance in its gaseous form gives rise to a coloured spectrum consisting of a number of very closely packed coloured lines. These lines form a pattern that is only created by that substance and this colour spectrum is the unique signature of that substance vibrating in a pattern of light frequencies. This is how we can detect different materials on distance stars for example.

The proportions of a substance's vibration patterns can be transferred to vibrating patterns of the clathrate micro-structure of water, provided that the appropriate section is available within the clathrate structure and a transfer structure exists.

When any substance dissolves in water it comes into a very intimate connection with the water micro-structures and they provide the transfer medium, or the speakers if you like, by which the vibration or information is transferred to other substances/cells within the body.

## HARMONY

Now all living structures are made up of a vast ocean of vibrations which harmonically interlock with one another. Life is in fact a product of harmony and, rather like when an orchestra plays a complex chord, there are a multitude of frequencies which take into account all the instruments and all their individual harmonics. If just one instrument plays a wrong note then the whole musical chord becomes discordant. This is through our experience of the disturbance in the ratio pattern of the frequencies.

Vibrating patterns are very powerful in organic processes. When they are correctly tuned to the organism's need, they harmonise and heal. If they are discordant they can cause considerable damage.

Water is a carrier of vibrating patterns, which are patterns of information that can be of use to an organism if they are harmonic. These patterns contain many frequencies in a particular proportion to one another and their pattern is a pattern of proportion or ratios held stable in the micro-structure.

Such structures are physically very small, but they're quite specifically ordered and very persistent, with patterns of immense variety. The primary source of these patterns is physical substance.

So that when water comes into contact with a physical substance or with any other force capable of imprinting vibrations on to its micro-structures (like a magnetic field for example) it takes on a memory of that physical substance or force. Since all organic tissues are formed through the agency of substances dissolved in water (and are therefore continually poised on the edge of being dissolved by the body's fluids) they're capable of taking on these vibrations into the clathrates/micro-structures of the water bound within their cells.

### RESONANCE

Imprinted water passing outside of a cell and having a strong resonance picked up from another force or substance elsewhere, can transfer this energy to water clathrates bound within the cell by the phenomena of resonance. Resonance here is defined as the free transfer of energy or the sympathetic vibration between one system and another without loss. Resonance is the function of mutually precisely harmonically related frequencies.

The balance between health and ill-health depends on the degree of harmony or discord set up in the micro-structure vibrations of water — the water that we drink.

## CHAPTER SIX

## *FOOD ENERGY*

The food supply we eat can give us energy but it can also take it away. There is an equation involved here between the amount of energy we can derive from a given volume of food, versus the amount of energy it costs our bodies to digest it. This is partly a function of the quality of the food we eat i.e. its food/nutrition value, and of its enzymic activity. For instance if we try to exist on a diet of cold, hard boiled eggs, we would do very poorly since they take a lot of energy from the body in the process of digestion. Whereas if we lived solely on ripe fruit we'd do very well because ripe fruit takes very little energy to digest. The crux of the matter of energy levels in food is enzymic activity. This again is a function of energy at the electronic/molecular level and here is how it works:

> All living organisms are (at a molecular level) integrated successions of enzymic reactions, and enzymes are charged protein molecules. These charged protein molecules act upon other substances, chemicals or by-products (these are called substrates) and change them whilst remaining unchanged themselves. Enzymes change substrates by splitting apart their molecules to form different substances as a product of that reaction, and under certain circumstances they can replenish their own energy in the process.
> 
> They split apart the substrate molecules in such a way as to ready them to become part of other protein complexes. This function is a bit like taking part of an electric circuit out and preparing it for use in a different circuit. The point being that the part taken out has a certain potential and as part of a living structure, retains a tiny living charge. That living charge is what makes it useful to the cells of the body as fuel and that charge is what is recognised and accepted by the immune system, as we shall see.

In the same way as the clathrate structures in water have a natural vibration, all other structures have a natural vibration which is the result of the atomic resonance of their component parts.

## THE FORCE OF LIFE

The force of life, the life force gives an extra dimension to the vibration of these structures, as we shall see in the final chapter, and this extra dimension is recognisable by other living structures which are capable of receiving energy from it by the function of resonance, as we saw in Chapter Four.

## VITAL RESERVES

Enzymes are produced by all the tissues and cells of the body and perform the function of distributing energy around the body by catalysing waves of energetic reactions between substrates that would otherwise remain inactive. We are all born with a certain/given level of enzymes in our body — our own vital reserves. If we live on a diet that continually challenges and depletes this enzyme reserve, then we become ill and die, whereas if we live on a diet that is enzyme rich and therefore adds to and maintains our natural enzyme reserve, then we stay healthy and live longer.

Once again it's a matter of energy input and use, which governs health.

Every living/organic substance has some degree of enzymic activity and these enzymes are transferred from one living system to another when we eat them.

## DEAD FOOD

Enzymes are unable to withstand high temperatures such as those used in cooking. As a result of this enzymes are completely destroyed in all foods that are canned, pasteurised, baked, stewed, fried or roasted. At 129 degrees Fahrenheit all enzymes are destroyed. Baked bread contains no enzymes neither do most butters which are pasteurised. Canned juices have minerals and vitamins, but the heating processes used in its manufacture kill the enzymes. Roasted breakfast cereals are devoid of enzymes and in fact heating at 60 degrees centigrade up to 80 degrees centigrade for as little as half an hour completely kills any enzymes.

Effectively cooking destroys all electronic activity in food and "shorts out" all its enzyme charges.

The protein molecules remain the same but they've lost their "life charge" they have no enzymic activity. They are dead!

If we then eat this cooked food we are importing into our body's large quantities of protein molecules which have little or no electronic activity. In order for these to be useful to the body they have to be "bump started". They have to be reactivated. This takes energy and the only place this energy can come from is the body's own enzyme reservoir.

So when we eat cooked (denatured) food our body's immune systems recognise this as completely lacking in electronic activity or natural energy potential, and react to rectify this situation. The white blood cell count increases and the white blood cells transport enzymes from all over the body to "combat" the problem of the energy sag caused by the dead food.

Enzymes are the scavengers in the body where they latch on to foreign substances and reduce them to a form the body can use or dispose of. When they are pulled away from their tasks, to deal with some other challenge elsewhere, then an integral part of the immune system is weakened and energy or vitality sag occurs throughout the body.

## THE FOOD CHAIN

To understand clearly how this happens we must look at what food does when it enters the body.

First though let's look at the structure of the body again:

It's common to think of the stomach and intestinal tract as being inside the body but for the purposes of food absorption this is not the case. The function of the entire digestive tract is to break down, process and in some cases rectify food products and bacteria taken in at the mouth, into a form which the body can use. Once this process has taken place then these energy rich products are passed through the wall of the gut and are carried by the bloodstream throughout the body, providing fuel for cellular activity. As we've seen in

Chapter One, the cells of the body use these complex sugars for their energy supply. There is no blood flow to speak of in the stomach or the gut and there are no blood vessels inside these organs for that purpose. All the food/fuel supply must first be transported through the walls of the bowel and the gut before it becomes available to be carried by the bloodstream to each cellular community.

### THE DOUGHNUT

The whole digestive system is a bit like a hole in a doughnut. If you put your finger through the hole, it is going "through" the doughnut but not through the substance of the doughnut. This is very important to an understanding of the role that food plays in health since a lot of mistaken ideas proliferate about toxic absorption through the bowels etc. Basically what is inside the bowel is outside the body. A healthy bowel wall is designed to resist the absorption and reabsorption of toxic materials. It is perfectly healthy for the body to contain discarded and decaying food waste and it's equally natural for the bowel to contain certain broken down and discarded body disconstituents. The bulk of healthy faeces is not "body waste" it is food waste taken in earlier at the mouth plus various discarded bacteria residues. It's not eliminated body waste because it's never been part of the body.

Left to its own devices, for example during a fast, the human gut is quite capable of breaking up all germs, viruses, bacteria and parasites, and will ultimately achieve a state of natural, healthy, odourless sterility PROVIDED IT IS NOT CONTINUALLY STUFFED!

We'll come to this question of over-eating later since it puts an appalling strain on the enzymic system.

### THE CATABOLIC RATE

We've seen earlier that the body is an interrelated harmonic energy lattice of extreme complexity and it's axiomatic that if we try to drive one of its systems too hard then we're going to

cause it and its associated systems to break down quite rapidly. In this context as Seneca said:
"Man does not die: he kills himself".
(By over-eating the wrong food!)

Life runs its course in direct proportion to the catabolic rate. The catabolic rate is the rate of tissue breakdown which is in direct proportion to the ageing process. Tissue breakdown is performed by enzymic reactions. The faster the enzymes are used up, the faster the breakdown. Our enzyme reservoir is the store of our body's vitality, its life force.

### THE "NUB" OF NUTRITION

We are born with a given component of enzymes (this is not necessarily fixed as we shall see, but it is what we start out with). These enzymes are living charges contained in various protein molecules which enable them to do work. Their work is to transmute substances taken into the body into fuel for the cells and tissues of the body to use. To do this enzymes break down or alter the configuration of food molecules rendering them useful to living systems.

### LEUKOCYTOSIS
#### (Increased White Blood Cell Count)

Our white blood cells are responsible for destroying disease-producing substances in the blood and lymph in the body. During acute diseases and infections the white blood cell count increases to help fight off these pathologies. White blood cells produce and transport enzymes throughout the body. At any time when the white blood cell count is increased to any extent, it is considered that an acute illness or infection is present somewhere in the body.

### INCREASED ENZYME COUNT

During acute diseases, enzyme levels rise. During chronic diseases, the body enzyme level is decreased. The pancreas and digestive system are in a weakened state and the immune system show signs of great expenditure. Thus enzymes are related to all diseases through the immune system.

### COOKED FOOD

When we eat cooked food white blood cell activity is increased and drawn into the gut area. This is because substantial quantities of protein molecules having no enzymic activity are being absorbed through the gut walls into the bloodstream and are placing a load on the enzyme system which is unable to cope. If these inactivated/non-living protein molecules are allowed to flood the system, because they have no electronic activity, they will rob the system of vitality by further depleting it of electrons. They will also begin to ferment in the bloodstream. Fermenting clumps of protein molecules are able to rob healthy cells of their electron charges and represent a dangerous catalyst to illness in the body. They can also form toxins which migrate to the tissues and joints of the body and also to fatty areas of the body where they're stored to cause trouble later. (See Healing Crisis Chapter Nine).

Accordingly the body musters all of its enzyme reserves to counter this threat. In populations where regular large quantities of over-cooked food form a large part of the diet, then cancer and other dread diseases are increasing at an exponential rate simply because the immune systems of the populus are being over-stretched on a regular basis. This continual stressing leads to the exhaustion of the immune system, to an overall dramatic reduction in vitality, and to premature death through a variety of life-style related diseases.

### FEAST AND FAMINE

Our hunter gatherer ancestors were almost constantly on the move and were perfectly adapted to long periods of relative privation interspersed by occasional "blow-out" feasts.

Feasting was to them an occasional treat (rather than the daily occurrence it is to us) and their stomach's were rarely stuffed with food. They were culled by the rigours of natural selection and were vigorously healthy with a keen understanding of the role that food played in their moods and make-up. They did not suffer from the diseases of modern man and by and large that was because they did not overeat and lived almost entirely on fresh food.

Their diet was largely made up of fresh ripe fruit, fresh ripe nuts, fresh ripe berries, fresh ripe vegetables, fresh growing shoots and fresh sprouting greens. Plus fresh ripe spring water! Their good food gave them life, health and strength by importing vitality into their bodies. Here's how:

### KIRLIAN PHOTOGRAPHY
(Electro-luminescent discharge from organisms)

Electrons are continually emitted from and absorbed into the body of a living organism as we've seen in Chapter Three. These electrons can be dissipated in a photographic emulsion in the same way as light. (In other words we can photograph them). An image is formed in the emulsion, dependent on the strength of the emitted electrons. And this image gives us a unique indication as to the degree of electronic activity present in any given substance. The degree of electronic activity in a living substance depends to a large degree on its degree of enzymic activity and so, using Kirlian photography, we can measure the levels of activity or life force in the food we eat.

Using this method it can be shown that as any growing food plant begins to ripen, its electronic and enzymic activity increases. The drive towards ripeness is a process of maturing in which the plant is involved in preparing ever more complex sugars from its component molecules.

This enzymic activity increases with increasing ripeness to the point where the fruit reaches a peak of activity producing complex short-lived sugars which contain vast quantities of bio-available energy. If this is then eaten by humans the maximum amount of energy is imported into the body and this is accompanied by the maximum number or quantity of highly active digestive enzymes. This predigested living food does not rob the body of enzymes in the process of digestion and places no consequent strain on the immune system.

### OUR TRUE LIFE SPAN

A live food diet of this kind is a great step toward full health. Animals that are not influenced by human beings have a perfectly healthy life, and almost all mammals have a life span of up to seven times their natural growth period. For human beings this would mean a life span of about 140 years of good health as opposed to the fore-shortened three score years and ten which have been our lot since we began to practise agriculture and cooking.

Further yet are the 40,000 chronic and degenerative diseases that are known in human medicine today, only around five are known in wild animals (who don't eat cooked food).

### QUANTITY VERSUS QUALITY

It's very clear from all the ancient Old Testament, and other pre-settlement texts which are still in existence, that we were once a very long lived species indeed. However the development of agriculture meant that we could dry and store our food surpluses and this brought about the need for extensive cooking to tenderise and reconstitute the food in an acceptable form. The consequence of this has been a proliferation of diet-related illness accompanied by a quite dramatic shortening of life-span and reduction in vigour!

CHAPTER SEVEN

## *ELECTRICITY, MAGNETISM AND ELECTROMAGNETIC ENERGY*

All life on earth evolved against a background of electrical, magnetic and electromagnetic fields which are forms of radiation affecting or having an influence on a particular region of space.

Electrical fields are fairly localised and don't spread out in space. They're quite easily screened against and don't penetrate many materials or organisms, generally only having an effect on their surfaces. When they vibrate they generate electromagnetic fields. Electromagnetic fields are always vibrating and always spread out into space indefinitely. They carry alternating electric and magnetic vibrations creating a dynamic "leap-frogging" matrix of concentric electric and magnetic fields. Whilst they can be screened out of small spaces their degree of penetration of materials depends on the frequence of their rate of vibration.

Magnetic fields can be static or vibrating. They are localised and do not spread out into space. They penetrate all materials and organisms and are very difficult indeed to screen against. When they vibrate they generate electromagnetic fields.

### EARTH'S FIELDS

Earth's electric field reaches from ground level up to the ionosphere about 100 miles up. Between the earth's surface and the ionosphere there is an electrical tension of between 200,000 and 300,000 volts but since there is almost no power in this field almost no-one is aware of it and no "shocks" can come from it.

However it's a very important source of power to living systems because it vibrates over a range of quite low frequencies. These frequencies occur between one and 30 hertz and are called the "Schumann waves". They have a pronounced peak of activity at about eight hertz and the human eye oscillates at several frequencies between eight hertz and 30 hertz thus enabling us to see. Further yet "Schumann waves" form the contour of human brain wave patterns in the alpha beta delta theta wave forms of electrical activity in our heads.

### SUPER-CONDUCTOR

As we've seen earlier the human body is made up of up to 90 per cent water which has some very interesting electromagnetic properties. This water has a high saline content which makes it a very good conductor of electricity and the cerebrospinal fluid is made of almost pure vitamin C which is an extraordinarily good conductor of electrons. Finally the brain is made up of totally unsaturated fatty proteins so that it behaves as an organic, body temperature super-conductor. There being no resistance to the passage of currents through its medium.

The whole structure of our bodies and particularly the brain-spine complex act as a perfect biological antenna conducting these resonances in the earth's electric field, throughout our structure enabling us both to see, also to experience different states of mental activity in harmony with our environment.

### COHERENCE AND CHAOS

As we've seen in Chapter One the life force uses every single possible energy source in its drive toward ever greater complexity and earth's electrical field is simply another example of this.

Living systems developed against a totally chaotic blizzard of extremely low frequency background electromagnetic radiation. They did this by organising around focal points where chaos confined itself to forms which, taken together, can be predictable. These are called fractals. The best example of this is a note on the musical scale.

A musical note is actually the product of a great variety of harmonics. These come together quite chaotically to form a difference frequency which is a pure note. Once they form that note they tend to go on doing so. This is because the overall note is itself stronger (more organised) than its component parts. It mode-locks or entrains them into a set pattern — a coherent pattern. The various components don't disappear and can re-emerge as chaos as soon as the dominant note dies away. The human body is made up of a vast number of systems which are the result of billions of different chaotic and quite random sub-systems.

### MAJOR SYSTEMS

Each of the major systems then is simply the physical expression of huge ranges of chaotic energy input, both from within the body and from without. Some of these come and go. They switch on and off, or fluctuate over predictable ranges. But the main system trundles happily on regardless, as long as it has an adequate level of energy input.

It hunts up and down as dominant factors in the energy input migrate up and down, but basically it stays within a given, if unpredictable range. The "main system" response is very important to health as it is the "ordering" force which results from chaos.

Earth's electrical field with its blizzard of varying systems is picked up and utilised by the human body as part of the "organising force" and is used to drive the brain waves and sight ability of our species.

### THE TRANSFORMATION

The key to the transformation of electricity into magnetism is vibration. If either one vibrates it turns immediately into the other and back again repeatedly, as described earlier. These electromagnetic fields have always existed on earth driven by every flash of lightning and, as we've seen in Chapter One, it's from the early flashes of thunder and lightning that life derived its first organising energy. When the elementary amino-acids were clumped together by the spiral vortexes of force created both by the impact of lightning on to the water of the vast early seas, and by the vibrations caused by the rolling waves of thunder in the water, these clumps formed the first of life's cooperatives.

The vortices being created basically by the flow of direct electric current (the flow of electrons) formed a left-handed pattern because direct electricity will only create a left-handed magnetic field. These left-handed structures form the template of life and, over eons, gave the spiral DNA its left-hand double spiral form.

### CHIRAL FORMS

Everything in creation has a mirror image and all amino- and nucleic-acids come in both left-handed and right-handed forms. Whilst these two forms are chemically identical in the sense of being formed from exactly the same atomic constituents, the chemical actions of the two are quite different, as a result of their being twisted in opposite directions by different spiral forces at the time of their creation. Throughout the universe there are similar numbers of left-handed and right-handed molecules, or molecules with their mirror images. Yet all forms of life use exclusively left-handed amino-acids to form proteins, and right-handed nucleic acids to form the genetic material of life. Living forms settled exclusively on L (evo) amino-acids and D (extro) nucleo-tides leaving out their mirror images. Their mirror images whilst having the same chemical form have different properties. They smell different, taste different and perform differently in chemical reactions from their left-handed (living) opposites. They are not capable of being integrated into living structures without first their molecular structures are altered back to left-handed again. This fact has considerable significance in relation to disease in our new, artificially created electromagnetic environment, as we shall see.

### NORTH-SOUTH POLARITY

If you blind-fold a hundred people, spin them round to disorientate them and then ask them to point to magnetic north, a statistically significant number of people will get it right. Clearly at some time in our evolution we had a use for this ability, probably using it, as the birds still do, to guide our migrations.

This planet's magnetic field which we sense, covers the entire surface of the earth, penetrates all the crustal rocks and the oceans and extends far out into space drawn out in a long magneto-tail away from the sun, by the force of the photon wind.

The variations in this field as it affects life on earth, have a number of frequencies embedded within them. They have a daily wobble as the earth rotates in its annual journey around the sun, also a cycle time of 24 hours due to this rotation. There is a 29 day cycle related to the phases of the moon, a 365 day cycle from the earth's relative annual movement to the sun. There are various cycles related to sun-spot activity which is driven by the sun's magnetic field folding in on itself and winding up to create huge magnetic storms on the sun's surface every eleven years. There are also many measurable variations which come from the inter-planetary magnetic field. Thus the earth's magnetic field is far from steady and undergoes both cyclical and apparently random variations of up to 2 per cent of its steady average value.

The steady average value of the earth's magnetic field is between 40 to 70 micro-teslas, depending on location. (A tesla is a unit of measurement of magnetic fields named after Nicolai Tesla). And it is this field that guides the needle of a compass.

Birds navigate and bees forage using sensory apparatus they've evolved which is capable of detecting magnetic fields around one nano-tesla, which is 50,000 times weaker than the earth's field strength.

Further yet the human pineal gland, which is one of the key organs of the body's hormonal/glandular regulatory system, has a magnetic sensitivity of 0.24 nano-teslas (200,000 times weaker than the earth's magnetic field). As we've seen already the earth's magnetic field is not steady but undergoes cyclical and apparently random variations. These variations are 1,000 times larger than the minimum for a bee to notice and register as a distinct change of state in the human pineal gland (and accordingly to hormonal levels in the human body).

This indicates that we unconsciously sense and respond to variations in the earth's magnetic field.

ORGANIC POLARITY

As far back as 1964 L. Gross showed that a small difference in a magnetic field can produce physical effects: magnetic fields modify the wave functions of electrons in macro-molecules, producing a greater para-magnetic susceptibility, which leads to a slow down in reaction speed, and the rate at which RNA and DNA are synthesised.

In other words, the replication of DNA macro-molecules is mediated by the action of the fluctuation in the earth's magnetic field, or DNA is very sensitive to magnetic fields.

DNA turns perpendicularly to a magnetic field and its electromagnetic sympathy is implicit in its structure and behaviour. It is a left-handed spiral form.

An electric current stands at right-angles to the resultant magnetic field, and an electric current will only create a left-handed magnetic field, as we've seen. Only left-handed amino-acids occur in living structures and it is along these spiralling lines of force created by the earth's magnetic field that amino-acids first clumped together to form our early cellular ancestors — the pre-cursors/progenitors of our DNA.

Life forms are thus the product of a cooperation between the various energy states of existence twisted into matter by the vortex forces created by a direct planetary electric current and its resultant left-handed magnetic field. Or to put it more simply, life forms follow predominantly the left-handed form this being one of the first energy/organisational, sources available to IT in the beginning.

WHAT COMES NEXT

This fact is very important to what comes next because recent additions to the background fields of natural electrical, electromagnetic and magnetic radiation via our new electrical technology, have had the effect of increasing the intensity, range and geographical distribution of these vibrations across an enormous spectrum of frequencies in all three fields.

Modern electrical devices use alternating current almost exclusively. Three-phase alternating current was invented by Nicolai Tesla in around 1882 and is capable of carrying electric current over long distances very cheaply. Three-phase alternating current is generated by placing three coils of wire around a soft ion core and supplying a current to each coil out of synchronicity with the others. This is a bit like a roundelay in singing where three groups sing the same song but begin four bars behind one another. Done properly the result is harmonic and very powerful. It's the same with electromagnetism, a magnetic field of considerable power is created between the coils and this field rotates perpetually in a RIGHT-HANDED DIRECTION!

## OUR NEW ELECTROMAGNETIC ENVIRONMENT

We depend on electricity for almost everything. We live in a world which is increasingly run and organised through electricity. This has given rise to a multitude of electrical machines which have become part of the fabric of our daily lives. The use of computers, fax machines, televisions, central heating pumps, florescent lights, photocopiers, washing machines and a host of other equipment has created a huge web of electrical wiring in every house, factory, public building and office. This complex new environment can have serious effects on our general health and well-being.

This is because the method of power generation used in almost every electrical device or system in use on the planet today is creating artificial spiral vortex fields which rotate in the opposite direction to the ones which occur naturally and are used within living systems.

## UNNATURAL FIELDS

We've seen earlier that moving magnetic fields can cause changes in chemical reactions and it is the reactions caused by magnetic fields which are rotating contrary to the natural rotation of the body's fields, which cause electrons to move in an unnatural or right-handed pattern. This is the cause of electro-stress and many illnesses including cancer. We did not evolve with these fields, they don't exist in the strength which we now experience them in nature, and they can kill us if we don't shield against them.

### DNA OSCILLATORS

Genes are not static one-off groups of chemicals but are oscillators with coherent frequency properties which they gained in response to the changing electromagnetic environment in which they formed over the aeons of their (our) evolution.

An ordered set of oscillators will produce a consistent patterning of material and it will ensure that the formation of new structures will occur according to a definite time sequence. This is a function much like the formation of "Chladni" shapes mentioned earlier where the shape changes in response to the frequency of the signal passing through the oscillator.

These patterning and growth development instructions are essential for a living organism to be able to unfold in the womb through its early evolutionary forms on to its most recent adaptation.

An ordered set of oscillators or patterned antenna will also, driven by the same energy/stimulus, continue to create rhythmic patterns of activity throughout the organism thus maintaining the whole body in a healthy pattern/condition.

In the human system these patterns are of a left-handed nature, they are the result of the movement of force fields which initially organised amino-acids/matter into left-handed structures, and these left-handed forces continue to operate in a healthy body. When they are subjected to interference from fields rotating in the opposite direction, a breakdown in the signals can occur. Aberrant signals emanating from an oscillator in a disturbed pattern can bring about profoundly different growth instructions in single cells and this is nowadays a major stressor which can lead to cancerous states obtaining in the body. This is because the cells are receiving the wrong growth instructions from the DNA which is being stimulated by the wrong signals.

## ENTRAINMENT

If 20 transistor radios are tuned close to (but not on) exactly the same broadcasting station, the din is horrendous. If one radio is then tuned exactly on to the correct wave-length and the volume turned up, something remarkable happens. All the other radios creep up or down the band width until they are all tuned exactly to the main broadcast. This is entrainment. A state whereby the major tone vibrations, slowly but surely push the off-station broadcast into synchronicity with themselves.

## HOMEO-DYNAMICS

Naturally coherent bio-rhythms are made up of a huge range of sub-harmonies which are chaotic as we've seen. Chaos is the natural state of the physical universe and our bodily states naturally reflect this. They oscillate over wide and unpredictable ranges in their normal performance. So much so the underlying processes are clearly random. Chaos is healthy.

## UNNATURAL COHERENT INFLUENCES

A mechanically generated electrical current has a magnetic field at right-angles to it.

When a living system is subjected to such a mechanically driven electromagnetic field, this can cause severe problems. If the field is coherent (ie. if it fluctuates at a rhythmic frequency or wave-length), and if this frequency is close to one of the body's natural rhythms then the unnatural mechanical field can "drive" the body's natural field rhythms to synchronise with it or to entrain with it.

In this way it may synchronise with a sub-element in a major system and pull the whole system out of its normal range of fluctuations, or it may drive several systems of chaotically interrelated activity to collapse, to exhaustion.

ULTIMATE STABILITY

A coherent electromagnetic field which is not synchronous with normal bio-fields is also very dangerous to biological systems. Bio-logical systems rely on the huge information input of billions of dis-ordered sub-systems for their healthy function. Bringing order to a disordered system structure in this way can cause the ultimate stability. It can cause degeneration of the living system which simply isn't strong enough to continually battle against the effects of coherent mechanically generated fields and breaks down.

SUMMARY

Artificial electric fields, electromagnetic fields and magnetic fields have the potential to damage living systems in the following ways:

1. Radiation of a frequency high enough to ionise gases (ionising radiation) causes cellular mutation, sterility and some forms of cancer by interfering with the DNA.
2. Lower frequencies can probably over time have a similar effect by accumulating as aberrant vibrations in the "memories" of the micro-structures (clathrates) in the water bound up in the cells of the body to such a point where they begin to interfere with the "normal" instructions given out by the DNA.
3. By entraining the naturally occurring bio-rhythms in the body and driving these to exhaustion.
4. Mechanically generated magnetic fields affect us by setting up vortices in the water of the body (which is up to 90 per cent of the body's volume), which rotate counter to those vortices created by natural organic systems within the body. Micro-vortices in water which are set up by movement are imprinted with electromagnetic information by picking up the vibrations of these radiations in the cone of force at the wide flat surface of the vortex. This is then amplified and transmitted through the vortex to be recorded in the form of molecular resonance in the clathrate structures of water. Accordingly once these counter-clockwise vortices

are set up they can amplify and transmit the wrong chiral form of information so altering the chemical structure and toxicity of the body and thereby placing a substantial and confusing load on the immune system.

## CHAPTER EIGHT

## *MIND*

Mind is the overall arbiter of health and is both the filter and the control by which the higher life forces organise the numerous systems within the body to repair and maintain themselves.

Streams of forces which have their origin outside the body are directed in their flow through the body by patterning and organising localised field forces which are influenced and controlled directly by the mind. To understand how this works it helps to think of a pond where two rocks have been dropped simultaneously on to the surface. Two sets of ripples flow out from the points of impact and where the ripples meet a completely separate pattern is set up. The rate at which this pattern vibrates is known as the "difference frequency" and is the product of the collision of the two sets of ripples. This is how it works in the human body — forces flow through it as we've seen, and these are acted upon and affected by systems of force or force fields set up in the body by its own internal activity, thus producing difference frequencies between the two. These difference frequencies like all other forms of available energy, are used by the body as a power supply.

### MOODS

This power supply is mediated by mood changes which, being capable of altering the hormonal balance of the body, are able to regulate and affect the degree of activity in its different cooperative structures.

### THE MIND-BRAIN-ENZYMIC RELATIONSHIP

One way we can see this at work is to look at the brain-mind-enzymic relationship. Nourishment of the brain with sugar and oxygen is the main priority of the human body. A drop in blood sugar can cause mental fatigue and depression. This can result in a substantial lowering of mood or, put another way, a change in the flow of emotions and a level of activity of the thoughts which flow through the mind.

As the sugar level drops, the metabolism of every organ drops.

Sugar levels in the body are controlled by the endocrine glands, especially the pituitary, the adrenals, the thyroid and the pancreas.

To remedy a drop in blood sugar, the pancreas secretes insulin which causes a further decrease in the sugar levels in the blood. Insulin moves glucose out of the blood into the cells. It also stimulates the liver and muscle cells to convert the stored carbohydrate glucose into glycogen. The adrenal glands secrete a hormone called epinephrine to break down glycogen into glucose which then enters the blood thus raising its sugar level again.

The thyroid gland secretes hormones that control the rate at which the body uses oxygen, its hormones also increase the rate of energy released from carbohydrates and so on.

These glands are all controlled by the pituitary gland which in turn is controlled by the area of the brain called the hypothalamus. The hypothalamus is actuated by, amongst other things, the emotions. So in this way the moods and emotions of the mind operating via the glandular system and neuro-hormonal activity are able to control the levels of activity throughout the body. In this way our minds mediate the healthy function of all the interrelated systems in the body switching them up and down in a continual pattern of adjustment to suit our different moods.

### TWO CENTRES

Mental activity has its focus in two centres of the body, the brain, and the stomach via the solar plexus. The human brain divides basically into two parts, the neo-cortex and the sub-cortex. The neo-cortex is the relatively recently developed area of the brain folded like a walnut around the older stem of the much earlier sub-cortex.

The neo-cortex is the focus of the main brain activity consciousness, with conscious control over a wide range of higher mind functions and it operates primarily through the nervous system receiving the bulk of its sensoral input through the sight organs in the head.

The sub-cortex is the repository of the earlier basic survival emotions. It's rather poorly linked to the neo-cortex with relatively few neuronal connections and this early brain structure receives a good deal of its information via the vagus nerve directly from the solar plexus.

Whereas the neo-cortex is informed and receives a huge part of its data input from the sense of sight, the sub-cortex receives its information from the senses which developed earlier, from smell, feel and above all from low frequency sound vibrations (most of which are too low for the ears to pick up) which are picked up and transmitted via the solar plexus and diaphragm.

These different sets of sensors link into different areas of the brain with which they developed in response to a particular level of our evolution.

Whilst all senses are ultimately arbitrated by the higher brain functions, nevertheless each of the senses informs a specific part of the brain and stimulates different forms of bodily responses.

For example, long before we developed sight, we developed smell, and our sense of smell (and taste) links to a very primitive area of the brain where it stimulates the very basic emotions which developed early in our evolution.

As we became more aware of ourselves and our environment, a process which took its great leap forward with the development of sight, we were required to use more sophisticated responses to more complex stimuli than those provided by our basic survival emotions.

We learned to focus, to concentrate, and with this function came cognitive intelligence, intuition and the ability to see into the future, to plan outcomes.

THE SOLAR PLEXUS

The solar plexus is located at the back of the stomach on a level about three inches above the navel, against the spine.

This organ is the main receptor and sensor of all of the range of vibrations emanating ultimately from the sun which our bodies use in a multiplicity of living functions.

The sensitivity of the diaphragm to tension is part of this process and historically we have been equipped to receive and utilise huge amounts of survival data through this organ complex. It acts as a sort of early brain system and was clearly developed in response to the need of our cellular cooperatives to react to ever more complex information from our environment as we developed. The development of the sub-cortex is directly linked to the functioning of this organ and this complex still plays a very important part in our lives and maintenance of our health.

UNITY AND FOCUS

The interconnection of the two brain systems into something resembling unity has endowed our species with an unique ability! This ability is a function of consciousness — the ability to focus.

The ability to focus our consciousness seems to be an unique human function in the mammal world, and the act of focusing is an act of control — a conscious function which can be learned and improved upon.

The ability to control our thoughts and emotions with practice, gives us the ability to control our health!

This is how it works:

> We generate about two million new blood cells every second. If we have a positive attitude to life, if our mind-fix or mind-set is dominantly optimistic and cheerful we increase our white blood cell corpuscle production. This is possible because when relaxed and happy we generate activity in those areas of the brain which are responsible for a clear optimum flow of energy through the body.

HARMONY

Let's look at this in another way:

If the brain-body complex is relaxed and under no stress, then it has within its blood supply an optimum balance of hormones for its healthy function, and will perform in close harmony with its environment. Harmony is the optimum level of activity where a clump of frequencies can best fit into a larger unity of frequencies passing through it, so as to be able to derive the maximum synergy with that system. A tone ment!

However the moment a negative thought or emotion intrudes, the body's systems immediately align or adjust themselves to deal with some perceived threat or stressor, then the whole hormonal balance changes and with it changes the conductivity of the various components of its make-up. The structure goes out of harmony with the forces of the universe and shifts to a lower level of health function efficiency.

Thus our dominant mood or mind-set mediates our health to a very high degree and this mood-related health is a function of harmony. Harmony in human kind is a function of the balance between our emotional brains, our intellectual brains and our physical environment.

THE BALANCE

That we exist on the spiritual, mental and physical planes is obvious. The spiritual plane of consciousness is that higher plane organised by the vast unconscious mind of the Universal Creative Intelligence as it is drawn down into physical reality through the upper vortex. This spiritual plane of mind is the organising force of all of the higher energies which flow down through each individual and without which there would be no life.

In the course of our normal lives we are not usually aware of the involvement of this level of mind, nevertheless it is the forerunner and form that all the energies which cascade through us throughout our lives will take. It is the vital spark.

The next level of mind is the conscious mind. The one which we use to think creatively and purposefully when we put together all of the ideas and impressions passed up to us by the subconscious.

The conscious mind is actually a bit of a misnomer because it flicks on and off quite rapidly as we go in and out of the fugue state (the daydreaming state) which is our normal mode of existence.

This conscious mind is what makes us human. It gives us the ability to focus our thoughts in such a way as to organise our lives and prioritise our habits.

When we concentrate we can make our conscious thoughts into things which will occur in our lives and this is because it informs and directs the subconscious mind.

The subconscious mind is the great engine, where all the primal drives and instincts live. This is the one that directs our daily lives and allows us to go through life on "automatic pilot", not having to concern ourselves about remembering to breathe or think about walking (or for that matter think about driving once we've learnt how) because it puts all of these functions and millions of others on automatic.

The conscious/subconscious complex can be likened to the captain of a ship directing the engine room. The captain (when he's on the bridge, or not in the fugue state) directs the engine-room as to what power is required and which rudders are to be used etc. The engine-room which is blind to the outside world, carries out these instructions faultlessly and to the letter. If the captain forgets to countermand an instruction then the engine-room is quite capable of driving the ship on to a reef, and this is what happens in many people's lives.

Be careful of the thoughts you think because thoughts are things to the subconscious!

## THE FLOW

When these three functions work in harmony we enter THE FLOW. The flow (also sometimes referred to as the "zone") is that state of optimum activity one sometimes witnesses in top sports people who describe themselves as being so caught up in their favourite sport/occupation as to experience "a spiritual involvement with the flow of achievement". This is difficult to describe in simple language but suffice it to say that if we are sure of the purpose of our life, intellectually involved in that purpose and physically working towards that goal, with a positive feedback, then these three aspects of our being will be in total harmony with one another. Under these circumstances we will rarely fall ill no matter what our physical environment, whilst at the same time being able to reach levels of achievement which, in our normal waking state, are unattainable.

To understand how this integrated system works and can be intentionally brought into use we must first look at some of the structures of life's forms.

## PATHCURVES

There are two opposing vortices flowing through all living systems. Those that flow up from the planet below and those that flow down from the universe. These can best be observed in the rotational layout of the fir cone or in the bud of new plant growth or the double opposed helix structure within an eggshell.

These and many similar forms in nature all show the formative influence of two flows of force which have worked not only to bring each structure together in the first place, but also to continue to guide its development as it grows.

Now force will always flow along the line of least resistance and so it is axiomatic that these lines must be established as forms or flow patterns in the fabric of our universe. I say this because every living, growing thing, uses these shapes and forms in the development of its structure.

From ram's horns to trees, to the double spiral vortices of the ears, everything occurs in nature in a form which can be enclosed in a double spiral made up of two spirals travelling in opposite directions. Two intersecting cones of force.

These shapes in time and space dictate the growth patterns of all living forms and are known in mathematics as pathcurve forms. A pathcurve form is one where, with the input of energy, as the form expands, its shape and structure remain the same. Or put in technical terminology - a line defined in projective geometry that is invariant in a particular transformation.

These pathcurve forms were discovered at the end of the 19th century and are developed using projective geometry which is a way of calculating how time will flow through a form affecting its growth and development.

Watching the mathematical transformation when a pathcurve form is expanded and developed is the same as watching a bud or shell grow in nature.

### THE CREATION OF ENERGY

During recent research into the interface between electromagnetic forces and life forces, it was discovered that these pathcurve forms are capable of creating a vortex of energy around themselves.

(This echoes the distinguished French physicist Leon Brillouin's work where in an effort to make gravitational theory compatible with classical electromagnetics he had to invent a second gravitational vector for correspondence with the electric and magnetic vectors. Then using the classical formula for field density, he went on to show that any spherical positive mass must be enveloped by a negative energy domain).

Pathcurve forms can now be shown to be shapes which have the property of creating measureable moving forces in space around themselves.

If however, the pathcurve form (of an egg for example) is distorted, then no vortex appears, no flow takes place. So that we are drawn inevitably to the conclusion that it is these shapes, which expand and dilate in time, that are the causes of the vortex flow upon which all life is based.

But which comes first, the spiral energy flow or the pathcurve shape? Does the flow already exist and is it simply concentrated by the shape or does the shape cause the flow? This is the eternal chicken and egg question of higher physics and can only be answered by saying that one cannot exist without the other.

### INTERLOCKING VORTICES

The opposing flow double spiral moves over a surface which is egg shaped, bud shaped, fir cone shaped or shell shaped, and so on. Movement in opposing flow double spirals or interlocking vortices can take no other form if it is to be successful, if it is to continue to exist, to continue to flow, and therefore the shapes are a function of movement.

Clearly the shape affects the flow else there wouldn't be different pathcurve form shapes but that all these are contained within vortices of moving energy is now scientifically provable. These energy vortices over forms can assume quite complex patterns. And the set of vortices surrounding an egg for example show a ten-vortice pattern rising vertically above the central axis of the egg with a further set of ten vortices upside down on the same vertical axis. Both these sets of vortices penetrate the form meeting and blending together, but the stem of the upside down vortices do not extend above the upper surface of the form.

There are two more axes which also carry vortices and these are not on the vertical plane but inclined at a variable angle to the vertical varying between zero degrees to 90 degrees, where they are free to rotate independently in the horizontal plane around the vertical axis.

The complete picture of this particular pathcurve form with its vortices presents a very complex structure with subtle and variable dynamics. And the two flows of energy which are inclined closer to the horizontal plane and swing around the vertical axis move in very variable and alive patterns sometimes swinging several degrees in a minute and yet at other times staying relatively static for quite long periods. The movement of these two inclined axes has a dynamic almost musical quality of inter-penetrating rhythms and the whole system of vortices and their dynamics goes through patterns of movement that have short, medium and long-term variations. The time of the day month and year all affect these dynamic movements which are also related intimately to the movements and relative positions of the planets and stars.

LIVING ENERGIES

The human body is developed from a pathcurve form and displays a symphony of pathcurve forms in its make-up. The vortices and their dynamics which are associated with these pathcurve forms intimately relate to the water which forms up to 90 per cent of our structures and to the organic processes taking place inside any living organism. THEY RELATE THE LIFE FORCES TO THE PHYSICAL SUBSTANCE THROUGH THE MEDIUM OF FORM ACTING ON WATER AND IMPRINTING ON ITS STRUCTURES!

## TIME

Movement takes place within time and we know that time in the physical world moves from past to present to future. But that time flow only accounts for one of the directional vortices which shape or are shaped by pathcurve forms. The other vortex travels in the opposite direction over pathcurve forms. So that in the metaphysical dimension time must flow from the future to the past.

That it does so is clearly evidenced by the existence of pathcurve forms in time and space, since without these there would be no critical paths for lines of force (be they life force or electromagnetic force) to follow, and therefore no growth, no life.

Let's look at this another way:

> Let us say that magnetism is a force having a negative charge and it flows in a broad river from the future to the past in a great spiral. As it flows through the ether it acts as a cause which sets up an effect. Let's say this effect is electricity which has a positive charge and flows in the opposite direction from the past to the future in a great spiral. These two great inter-locking spirals flow through each other but in opposite directions and as they brush against each other they set up a difference frequency. This comes into physical existence continually as their forces spill into an area of turbulence, of ripples and eddies, of minor vortices. These form predictable stable patterns. This area of the inter-face of times flows, this difference frequency, is what we experience as physical form. In it everything vibrates at different speeds or rates. Some parts vibrate so fast as to appear solid and others less so, but all are created continually by the contra-flow of time.

## CAUSE AND EFFECT?

That there are two time-lines in action in opposite "directions" is exemplified by the fact that often what we see as effects can occur in advance of causes as well as vice-versa.

## PHYSICAL FORM

Physical form then is the difference pattern of the contra-flow of two forms of time, that which exists on the physical plane and that which exists on the spiritual plane.

This is simply another way of saying that any force moving in one direction sets up an equal and opposite force in the other direction and is an obvious extension of the law of cause and effect.

The movement of the past to the future is mirrored by the movement of the future to the past as follows:

You are born, grow up, live and ultimately your physical body dies — this exemplifies the flow of time from past to future. However in your mental life, in your mind, you can foresee events in the future, watch them come into being and then flow past you into their futures which become your past. In this way you can watch the opposing flow of time in action (although you can't actually physically experience it on this plane).

## TWO VORTEX

This ability of mind to conceive and observe the counter-flow of time is a function of the spirit, mind, body interface in human structures. The human body is a vast collection, a symphony of pathcurve structures. From the vortex which appears on the crown of the head to the whorls of vortex forms on the fingers and toes (fingerprints) the opposed double spiral, interlocking vortex is the pattern of our structures. The form of the neural canal can only be developed by two incoming opposing vortices and its only when these two opposing forces are acted upon by the two further vortices close to the horizontal which are a consequence of the pathcurve egg form, that the full pattern of the human living structure can develop.

The human egg as it develops into the embryo then is worked upon by two vortices coming from opposite directions. One, the physical, flowing from the past to the present, and one, the spiritual/mental, flowing from the future to the past. The closing up of the embryonic disc starts in the middle of the neural plate in an area which will later become the base of the neck and this pattern of growth is held to throughout the duration of life on earth.

### TWIN CONES

Because of this process of formation the human head becomes the seat of consciousness and knowledge. Here resides the ability to look forwards into the contra-flow of mental/spiritual time and observe events perceived in this way.

The trunk on the other hand formed by the earth vortex of physical time, is the region of the unconscious, the product of the accumulation of forward flowing time.

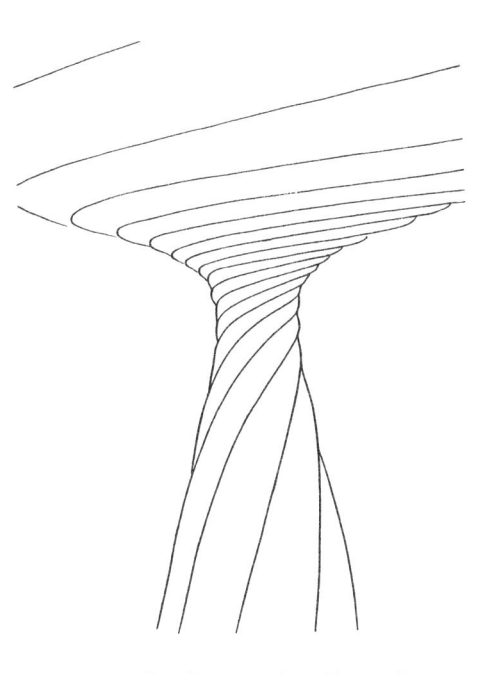

Fig 4 The Confluence of an Airy and a Watery Vortex

The human form then is seen as the confluence of two cones of opposing rotational force meeting with the tips or points in the area of the neck and shoulders.

### TWO POLES

The head area which is formed and influenced predominantly

by the vortex flow of time travelling in the direction of future to past, is the focus of the frequencies of a higher vibrational nature which penetrate into the body as the controlling or formative characteristics of its matter. The influence of the spirit.

Whilst the rising vortex of the lower physical form is the consequence of the upper vortex, brought into being and mediated by the existence and activity of the other. These vortices change direction of rotation in the neck area where they meet, and the cross-over point between the two is where the huge outflow of energy takes place which energy forms and flows into and over the human pattern.

Our ability to consciously adjust this flow of energy by altering components of the spiritual/mental vortex gives us the power to shape our health and our future as we shall see.

### THE PHYSICAL BODY

The physical body is the accretion of the difference pattern set up by the two energy vortices. Each of these vortices has what can be termed its own set of "sensors" by which it relates to the world in which we live, but the migration of intelligence to the use primarily of sight as our main sensory input has made for an increased ability to concentrate our attention in the upper vortex area.

This migration of senses into the area of the spiritual/mind related vortex, with the increased ability to focus on distant objects and interpret coming events, is what has given us the ability to consciously control our physical bodies through our mental processes.

This is the ability by which we can achieve harmony throughout our three different levels of being and this harmonic function is the mediator of all health.

### CONSCIOUS CONTROL

The conscious mind informs the subconscious which is how we learn and accumulate knowledge. The subconscious mind acts almost exclusively on the instructions it receives from the conscious mind and certainly always follows its most deeply held wishes and assumptions.

That the conscious controls the subconscious in this way can be demonstrated by the fact that Christian scientists who believe most profoundly in the power of prayer, are regarded as better risks by the actuaries of the insurance industry and given lower rates of insurance cost because they tend to live longer (they believe they will).

A better example is provided by the fact that old or ailing people will often wait until after Christmas or a visit by their loved ones before dying.

Or yet again that the rate of suicides falls off when there is a war on because people are bound up in a common purpose and joined in a common goal "which they believe in".

In each of these examples the consciousness of the group or people involved is a decisive factor in their will to live. These are all examples of conscious control over physical function.

THE PURPOSE OF LIFE

To fully understand the above we must look at the purpose of life. All time, matter, life, energy and consciousness began with the BIG BANG and expands outward from that event.

Spiralling outward from that event all force flows set up an equal and opposite flow which, when the outward spiral reaches the limit of its energy, will pull everything back in on itself to collapse into a black hole before the whole process begins again.

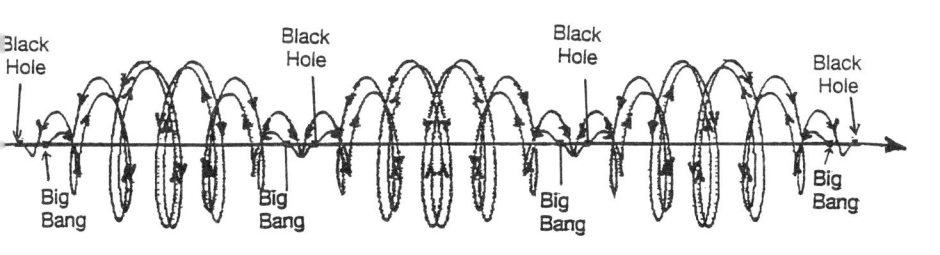

Fig 5  The Cyclical Wave Form Structure of the Universe

These two counter-flows are the counter-flows of time referred to earlier. This gives the universe a cyclical wave form structure as it flows outward and inward in the continual process of creation.

Because these spirals form "enclosing" vortices and flow in opposite directions they impart to the area contained within them, the pathcurve form of an egg. This is why this is the most preferred form in creation. But more to the point as the universe expands it moves out into ever greater volumes of space in which yet more "events" can occur. Each event is a cause and each cause an effect so that the universe becomes a vast store of information consequent on the number of events it experiences. As yet more events are stored in the fabric of the expanding universe it becomes sentient with the purpose of accumulating ever more information and experience.

This universally creative dynamic gives rise to a proliferation of living forms born out of the counter-flow of time energies, and these are imbued with the common purpose of the universe, which is to learn — to be creative.

As the universe itself evolves through countless such cycles it devises and develops multitudes of different levels and planes of existence through which its creations (or sensors) migrate. These form a series of levels of existence through which its learning functions progress.

The universal intelligence, possessed of a desire to create, to constantly seek new knowledge through the experience of all of its creations, is what is the motive force of all life.

Consequently to come into complete harmony with the life force we must be creative, be absorbed in the creative process.

Each human being is different from but similar to all others. Each has an important contribution to make to the ever expanding store of universal experience. Each is a part of that expanding universal intelligence and each part will develop and continue to be viable as a consequence of their conscious contribution to the growing knowledge and experience of the universal intelligence.

To put that in a different way, you will continue to be viable and healthy as a part of creation as long as you are contributing in your own way to the overall purpose of that creation.

As we will see in the conclusion there is only one definite sure-fire way of doing this. More of which later.

## SINGLE CURVES

The purpose of life is to learn, to develop and above all to be creative. This is the prime directive of the Universal Creative Intelligence because this ability, to develop, try out and discard billions of alternatives, is what dictates future events.

The Universal Creative Intelligence (which is all of us and all of the universe) focuses in the present instant. It is an accumulation of all the events that have ever taken place and is aware of all possible futures, because of the duality of time. But it is not yet formed of those future events which have not yet occurred.

The past is a pattern or a series of patterns that it created, and the future is a single curve (uni-verse) waiting to be created. Only human kind with its ability to see into the future, is able to know what can happen. Only human kind can predict what might happen, and only human kind with its ability to change conditions and adapt circumstances, has the ability to create what will happen.

This creative function obtains on an individual level as well as a species wide level and it gives us the ability to create our own personal futures, as well as those of our species and the others with which we are involved.

Let's look at that a different way:

> The ability to visualise a goal is a function of the focused conscious mind looking into the future. The conscious mind instructs the subconscious mind which makes that goal a priority for all the body's systems. The unconscious mind (which is the vast mind of the Universal Creative Intelligence) then sets about hardening the visualised goal into reality so as to progress/expand to new horizons (or if you like, so as to evolve through new learning).

The strongly visualised future becomes the chosen event, the new reality. The ability to choose the future is the purpose of human kind.

## LEARNED EVENTS

In the late 19th century glycerine came into use and whilst it was known that it could crystallise no-one was able to achieve this without a great deal of trouble. In the normal course of commerce a train load of glycerine was sent over the Alps and during its journey the glycerine on board was subjected to freezing temperatures and all manner of chaotic vibrations. Overnight it all crystallised out much to the surprise of all concerned. From that point on all over the world glycerine began to be easy to crystallise. The Universal Creative Intelligence had learnt!

Nowadays it's an accepted phenomenon in chemistry that often when you find or develop a new material, it will be difficult to get it to crystallise for the first time. But as time goes by it will crystallise with greater and greater ease (as a Universal Creative Intelligence remembers the new event).

## THE HUNDREDTH MONKEY SYNDROME

Similarly in mental terms there is a well known example of the half wild monkeys which inhabit several islands off the coast of Japan and spread over a small archipelago.

These monkeys were regularly fed sweet potato and whilst being observed in a scientific experiment which took place over several years, it was noticed that one of the senior female monkeys had taken to washing sweet potatoes given to her, in the sea. Initially this was probably to get the grit off them but later because she liked the taste of salt on them. She taught all of her off-spring and slowly the idea spread throughout her group, when all of the monkeys in that group began to take their sweet potatoes into the sea and wash them before eating them.

When this practice had reached a critical mass in the local monkey population it suddenly spread throughout the entire monkey population along the archipelago! The point being here that many of these islands, containing separate colonies of monkeys were divided by miles of sea and there was no visible method of communication between the monkeys from island to island. Nevertheless washing the sweet potatoes had become a learned response throughout the entire monkey population or in other words the Universal Creative Intelligence had learned.

This function of critical mass plays a very real role in informing the Universal Creative Intelligence and ideas (sometimes described as MEME's,) when observed to reach the critical mass are transmitted around the world becoming habit patterns and therefore stepping stones to future development.

This process of guided evolution is part of a process of positive feedback between the Universal Creative Intelligence and its sentient units/cells and has lead at different times and in different cultures to the concept of a personal individual God.

The vast unconscious "mind" of the Universal Creative Intelligence uses all "events" which come to it to guide its journey into its future creativity and a knowledge of this characteristic can be used to your advantage and to help you get better if you are ill, as we shall see.

## CHAPTER NINE

## *WHAT TO DO TO HELP YOURSELF*

To help your immune system to re-establish your normal healthy functioning it is important to do three things:
  (a) remove the stress on it which has made you ill.
  (b) help your body to function in a much more healthy way in future.
  (c) change your life — redefine your function in life so as to harmonise more closely with your purpose, (this time round).

### THE BEGINNING

None of the following suggestions taken individually will achieve any of these three priorities, but taken as a whole and integrated into your way of life, they have the power to dramatically change your health and the circumstances of your life for the better.

### VITAMIN C

We evolved as migratory omnivores taking in huge quantities of vitamin C as an integral part of our diet. In Chapter One we saw how vitamin C is vital to the healthy function of the human body, so it's very important to begin taking large quantities of vitamin C as a dietary supplement.

The human body can't store vitamin C so it should be taken throughout the day with water. When I became very ill some years ago, I began by taking 20 grams of vitamin C a day and from that point on I could chart my recovery. Now 20 grams may seem a lot but it was obviously needed and since the body can't store vitamin C this has to be sourced entirely from our daily diet, so the body is designed to take exactly what it needs and dump the rest.

This function is very useful and will help you to gauge how much you should take. Start with doses of 5 grams dissolved in water. Take this dose four times a day. (If you can't get any of the soluble vitamin C then buy the tablet form and take five of these with at least a pint of water four times a day). Continue this dosage until you get a loose bowel movement then back off to taking 3 grams each time, but increase the frequency of the dosage. In other words take 6 doses of 3 grams at equal intervals throughout the day rather than 4 doses of 5 grams. This way your body has time to absorb all it needs and will begin the repair process.

As you begin to mend you will continue to need high doses of vitamin C and you'll be able to adjust to your own particular optimum intake by using your bowel movements as a guide. If you are "over-dosing" on vitamin C you will be flatulent and have loose movements, but when you get it right you'll feel much better and have comfortable firm movements.

Please note that it is very important to your ongoing health that you continue to take vitamin C for your rest of your (hopefully long and healthy) life. To this day I take a minimum of 6 grams every day. It helps me, stay free from colds, suffer reduced stress, have a very healthy bowel, and never concern myself about cancer.

Vitamin C taken in high doses as a food supplement, (with food) is a vital catalyst to good health.

Vitamin C is a powerful antioxidant which means it mops up free radical molecules quite easily, thus reducing a whole number of stresses on your immune system. Because of this and the fact that your whole intestinal tract becomes more healthy, you will find that your complexion improves, your skin tone improves and you generally look and feel better.

As we saw in Chapter One vitamin C is the body's natural catalyst to electronically desaturate protein and make it more conductive to electrons, more vital! This being so you can expect to undergo an healing crisis during the first four to six weeks of taking mega doses of vitamin C.

HEALING CRISIS

This healing crisis is where you actually feel much worse for a short period. This normally begins two to three weeks after you start the high doses of vitamin C and lasts about four days. A healing crises is caused by the release of toxins stored in the tissues of the body. Here's why:

For years you have eaten unsuitable foods, that is to say, foods which we are not designed to eat often. As a result your system has been continually overloaded and has had to deal with quantities of toxins which it cannot properly process. It has dealt with these by depositing them in the tissues of the body where they stay, "furring up" your system, and creating an internal environment where illness and disease can find a fertile home.

For years your bowel and bloodstream have become more sluggish having had to deal with abnormally large quantities of proteins and fats. These have taken up all its dietary sources of vitamin C in order to process and use them as building blocks in the body. This has left you in a condition of hyperascorbemia — a chronic shortage of vitamin C. (This condition is very common in the West where a cooked food diet, very deficient in vitamin C, is all too often the "norm", and it is the reason that we heal so slowly and recover from illness so slowly in later life).

When you begin the regime I'm talking about, you suddenly reverse the process. For the first time in years you are now supplying your body with the catalyst it needs to process all the proteins and toxins its had to store in your bodily tissues. It can now begin to do this properly and it does so with a will.

As systems which haven't worked properly for years, begin to revive and come back into optimum function, all the stored waste, fats, toxins and half digested proteins are precipitated back into your bloodstream for reprocessing.

This usually causes spots, a feeling of lassitude and a whole range of minor illness symptoms, but it's a good sign because it simply means that your body is at last able to catch up on unfinished business and rid itself of a lot of stored poisons.

The healing crises will not harm you and is part of your general recovery. You can't begin to get properly better until you go through this, so don't worry. It's a good sign.

## PREFERRED FORMS

Once you begin to stabilise after this phase (or anyway after about four weeks of going on a high vitamin C intake) you will need to sort out your preferred form of vitamin C and find a good source of supply. I say this because it isn't cheap and is better bought in bulk and kept in the dining room on hand as a regular part of your new regime.

I began by taking large quantities of vitamin C in its soluble form because I was so ill I had difficulty swallowing tablets/pills. However once I got past the healing crisis and began to recover, I was able to swallow better and begin to plan for the future.

After experimenting with various types of vitamin C in pill form, I found the one which suited me best is a very simple compound of vitamin C with the bio-flavanoids with which it naturally occurs in growing fruit.

These bio-flavanoids have a catalytic action on the vitamin C and for me they made it more easy to integrate into my diet.

I now take four tablets with each meal with water, and I ingest them one at a time during the meal.

In my view vitamin C is misnamed as a vitamin — it's not simply a catalyst for the use of food in the body but is one of the main corner stones of healthy living.

In fact a lack of vitamin C causes scurvy which is a breakdown of the cohesive bonds within the body and amongst the early symptoms of scurvy are the opening of old wounds and an inability to heal simple scratches.

Scurvy was eliminated in the British navy during the 19th century by a daily ration of limes being handed out to the crew and this is where the American expression "limeys" comes from when referring to us.

A poor diet deficient in vitamin C will cause scurvy — a rich diet deficient in vitamin C will cause hyperascorbemia. Nowadays our diet is made up almost entirely of processed and cooked food and we all suffer from hyperascorbemia — a deficiency of vitamin C.

OVEREATING

According to the structures of our pallets and our gut, we have evolved to live on masses of raw fruit, shoots, nuts and vegetation with very occasional (and often dangerous) intakes of raw meat.

We are designed with digestive systems capable of getting the very maximum energy and food value out of a wide range of diets, and we are evolved to live well on very little food.

We clearly lived until fairly recently as hunter-gatherers, and the rhythms of such a life would have meant enduring long and regular periods of hunger. We are actually structured to respond to wide fluctuations in food supply and to go hungry or slightly hungry for much of the time.

During the Second World War, when I was born, the population of England as a whole had to manage on very simple rations, with little in the way of processed foods. They were far more healthy then than we are now (despite the appalling stresses and strains of total warfare) and its clear from this that most illness is diet related.

This is also clear proof if proof be needed, that almost any mental or physical stress can be borne almost indefinitely as long as the rule of simple and "spare" eating is observed.

FOOD STRESS

If your body is stuffed with denatured foods it has to work hard to process these and distribute/dump them round your bodily tissues. By altering your diet you can eliminate this stress and help your system back into full health again.

This is really hard to come to terms with, and at first it's going to take all your concentration and willpower to achieve, but you must EAT LESS! You should now eat about half of what you ate before.

Unless you are doing hard physical work you do not need to take in large amounts of food each day. On the contrary you need to take in, to eat, small amounts of the right food regularly, as we shall see.

Repeatedly in the last 3,000 years outstanding individuals have tried to tell the public about the relationship between food and health, but the public at large have obstinately resisted such teachings. Probably the best illustration of the link is supplied by the writings of an Italian nobleman, Luigi Cornaro of Padua who lived 400 hundred years ago. His lively wit and longevity make his work just as relevant today as it was when he wrote it and a broad overview of his story is as follows.

> "It is in everyone's power to eat and drink what is wholesome and avoid overfeeding. He that is wise enough to observe this will suffer little from other incapacities. The man who pursues a temperate life with all possible exactness will seldom, if ever, be seized with a disease".

He later wrote that after a riotous youth, by 40 he was broken down and said to be dying. His two doctors, with their medicines and unwanted food, he dismissed and resolved to overcome his intemperate ways. He is quoted then as saying "alas for my clever physicians - they are long dead, while I, age 100 remain in excellent health". His final and most pithy observation is "he who would eat much must eat little; for eating little lengthens a man's life, and by living longer he may eat a great deal more". Cornaro died at 102, absolutely without pain, sitting in an easy chair.

In a later generation George Bernard Shaw the great playwright provides a similarly good example. He had a poor body and suffered indifferent health but by abstemious eating he managed to maintain a virile mentality until the day of his death.

It's extremely hard to change dietary habits built up over a life time but in order to recover vigorous good health and maintain it for many years you must take charge of your own life and begin to redevelop your own sense of identity.

THE POISON INDUSTRY

Unfortunately there's a vast industry whose fortunes depend on persuading you to eat as much as you can whenever you want to. Another aspect of that same industry sells you billions of pounds worth of patent medicines and constipation "cures" to "help" you deal with indigestion and the other results of overeating.

Basically you are just the "mug in the middle" stuffing yourself so that they can profit and in fact killing yourself young by overeating the wrong foods in a frenzy of insecurity brought about by advertising which is by and large designed to play on very deep seated and unprotected biological imperatives.

The entire physical and mental health complex of an individual is mediated by what and how much they eat. You simply cannot be healthy if you eat large quantities of processed food regularly!

Processed and cooked food is denatured as we saw in Chapter Six. If contains very few or no enzymes and costs you a lot of energy to digest. That energy is drawn from throughout your body and leaves you weaker, more susceptible to illness. Also, and more to the point in this context, it leaves you less able to recover or fight back once you have an illness.

The correct healthy diet for human beings is ripe fruit, ripe nuts, ripe seeds, ripe vegetables, ripe salads, ripe vegetation and ripe water. (More of which later).

### JUICING

At the outset of my illness I didn't feel at all like eating but as my appetite returned and fluctuated I began to eat the fruit people had brought me. As time progressed I became bored with this alone and began to look for ways of expanding the range of my diet.

I reasoned that as well as eating less food in terms of bulk, I would also benefit from eating more energy-rich food and I finally struck upon juicing as a method of achieving a really good diet.

Drinking juice made from fresh ripe, enzyme rich food, puts little stress on the digestive tract and since juices are so easy to absorb, their nutrients go into the bloodstream in minutes.

This is a sharp contrast to the hours it takes to digest a cooked meal that is eaten, since the small amount of nutrients it yields often take hours to finally get through to the body. Moreover uncooked juice retains all the enzymes (food value) it has ripened to produce.

Juice made a remarkable difference! All of a sudden my body was getting fed with easy to digest liquid food with all its nutrients and enzymes intact. As my health continued to improve I began to feel more hungry between meals and I found that the best way to combat this was to juice and drink a couple pieces of fruit every two hours.

This stayed the pangs of hunger and by experimenting with different fruit complexes I was able to decide which suited me best.

This also opened the door to a vast range of tastes and flavours that I had experienced only "dully" before and made for a new form of "COOL COOKING" which I'll describe later.

By experimentation I found that I preferred fruit juiced in the mornings and vegetables in the afternoons and evenings. This is probably because oxygen released by vegetation continues up to mid-day and then switches to $CO_2$ absorption from then on, which tends to slow down enzymic reactions in fruit but favour those in root vegetables in the afternoons.

By the third month of this new diet I had invested in a very good quality juicer simply because I was juicing such a wide range of produce. It's not necessary to spend a lot of money to do this however as the same results can be obtained by putting the food through a blender and then pressing out the juice.

This has the added advantage than you can then eat the resultant pulp with ice-cream or yoghurt and it makes an excellent pudding.

ADJUSTMENTS

By this stage in my changed regime I was taking large

amounts of vitamin C, regular daily drinks of fresh juice and eating about half of what I used to eat.

I found that because I was eating primarily fresh fruit and vegetables, which have a high vitamin C content, I was able to drop back my daily intake of vitamin C to between 5 and 6 grams. I also found that the volume of my bowel movement reduced dramatically. This was because I had reduced the amount of food I had been eating, which in turn reduced the bulk of intake, the food I did eat being used much more efficiently.

As another beneficial side effect, I now notice that my food intake requirements fluctuated in direct proportion to the amount of exercise I was taking and my weight stabilised at a very healthy level leaving me leaner and fitter than I had been for 20 years. I was clearly moving toward my optimum diet.

## DIET

I then began to examine my main diet and concluded that although I had reduced my food intake, which had helped me to reduce the strain on my system, I could do more to convert my diet intake into one which would provide me with a series of more positive benefits. I was at that time a meat eater, but realising that this put a lot of very complex toxins through what was basically a vegetarian/fructivorian intestine structure, I began to look at the possibility of becoming a vegetarian.

First I examined ancient cultures to find out why meat had crept into our diet, and discovered some interesting facts. According to the Old Testament, much of which is derived from far earlier Sumerian writings, humans began life by eating only fresh fruit and vegetables. The ancient religion of Hinduism and in fact most of the religions stemming from the Far East and the Indian subcontinent (which spring from the non-violent stem of human philosophy), do not to this day eat meat. The Essenes an Israelite brotherhood (also known as the desert fathers) who lived on the shores of the Dead Sea beginning from about 200 years before the birth of Christ, appeared to me to have been carrying on Buddhist traditions which originated further east. They numbered about 4,000 in biblical times and maintain themselves by agriculture, holding all property in common and sharing each other's needs. They were highly religious, did not sacrifice animals and because, they believed in complete cleanliness of the body, dressed always in white. They were strictly vegetarian and Jesus of Nazareth, who was an Essene followed the vegetarian way throughout his life.

A misunderstanding has arisen here because when Jesus spoke of meat he was referring to food of a vegetarian nature. Greek is the language by which the Bible came down to us and the Greek word which we loosely translate as meat merely means food or nourishment. Thus Jesus didn't say "have you any meat" but "have you anything to eat"?

Jesus said "if you eat living food, the same will quicken you, but if you kill your food, the dead food will kill you also".

Essene children were taught the simple rudiments of faith in God, that they must do unto others as they would have the others do unto them, and above all, that work brought results.

A boy of twelve was at that time regarded as a mature individual who knew the natural laws of health and had been taught to realise that a clear mentality depends upon a clean, vigorous body.

### A SACCULATED BOWEL

Looking for further corroboration of a vegetarian past I found that uncivilised tribes living on a largely vegetarian diet are not afflicted with cancer any more than wild animals are, yet when these same tribesmen adopt civilised food (meat, eggs and milk etc) cancer develops. Much known information now corroborates this evidence but the chief fact is that flesh food often rots before elimination. So that putrefying residues are absorbed into the bloodstream from the colon poisoning the whole organism as a consequence.

This occurs a lot in humans because of the structure of the bowel. The small intestine is basically a long spiral tube with a series of sac like or egg shaped variations in its length. When it's stretched out this gives it the appearance or shape of a long necklace of small lumps and these sacs have a specific job to perform.

Raw vegetation or fibrous matter is often quite high in cellulose which is difficult for our digestive systems to break down and use. To facilitate the use of this food which, in our recent past, (up to about 10,000 years ago) formed our main diet, we evolved a sacculated bowel. This structure slows down the rate at which our food is evacuated and allows movement of the body to "massage" the lower abdomen so as to "work" or "kneed" the partially digested food as it passes through the intestine. (This why walking after a meal can help digestion).

However the sacculations in the bowel, evolved to aid in the digestion of simple vegetable and fruit material rich in its own enzymes, have just the opposite effect on meat. They slow it down dangerously!

All carnivors have smooth bowels. These enable them to eat fresh killed meat, full of the fear hormones like adrenalin, and very poorly supplied with natural enzymes. Their systems take what they need very quickly from this rapidly decaying toxic mass and then get rid of the residues very quickly through their smooth bowels, so as to avoid the bulk of toxic absorption.

They have evolved to have short, fast, aggressive lives, derived from the steady build up of toxins in their bodies, and they cannot easily live on any other form of food.

Humans on the other hand are omnivors and we have developed to live on a very wide range of diet the greater bulk of which has always been raw fruit and vegetable matter. Our bowels are designed to slowly "work" our food through our digestive system so as to be able to absorb the maximum amount of food value from the enzymic activity which continues to take place in the intestine.

Meat treated in this way quickly goes bad, becomes toxic and presents our bowels with a challenge. Once in a while this does little harm and our immune system rises to the challenge very well, but when the bowel has to deal with this situation repeatedly, as it does with our modern cooked meat and two veg diet, it ultimately breaks down and allows untreated toxins derived from the unnatural food in the bowel, to flood the body. This is the root cause of most illness!

In a study performed at the Harvard Laboratories of Physiology, it was shown that a meat diet produces an acceleration of the heart action that's surprising in its magnitude and duration. After a meal of meat the increase of the heart rate regularly amounts to between 25 per cent and 50 per cent more than its previous level and persists for 15 to 20 hours. This is a total of many thousands of extra heartbeats and its known that it requires the presence of internal poisons to cause the body's functions to accelerate in this manner. Thus the evidence of the presence of these poisons is the quickening of the body function.

I resolved to give up eating meat!

## FASTING

Realising that for years I had been eating my way to an early grave, I began to look for a way of thoroughly cleaning out my system. I noticed that throughout the history of religion and philosophy great emphasis had been placed on regular fasting as a method of clearing the mind and "purifying" the body. I examined the results of this and discovered an interesting capability that we humans share with several other mammals who hibernate.

If we stop eating for a time our bodies work away steadily and use up all the food matter available in our intestines. Everything is gradually broken down and used and this process continues until nothing is left. In this way all the cellulose and all of the other hard to use material, which would normally be ejected, is broken down and used, until the digestive system is thoroughly empty.

Then and only then does the body begin to use its reserves of stored fat and as these too are processed into glucose the toxins they often contain are dealt with by the immune system, often being excreted through the skin as perspiration.

Finally the bloodstream is cleaned of all toxins and foreign matter by the enzymes and white blood corpuscles and the body becomes completely healthy.

The bowel at this point becomes completely sterile!

This knowledge, derived from an observation of the hibernation habits of bears (and its correlation with various human experiments), led me to the conclusion that at some time we too had probably hibernated as a survival pattern. Or had at least developed a similar "housekeeping" pattern in our systems which came into operation during periods of what was probably annual privation in winter. This reflex can be used today to get back to full health and stay that way!

With knowledge of the foregoing it's axiomatic that the human body is perfectly capable of clearing up almost any illness if it's left to its own devices to do so and if all extraneous stressors are removed or reduced as far as possible.

I began to fast one day a week and in a very short time my overall health and digestion improved noticeably.

COOL COOKING

As I said earlier, I had decided to become a vegetarian but a vegetarian with a difference! I reason that if I switched from a cooked meat/fish and vegetable diet to a cooked vegetable diet only, I was still having to get my immune system (enzymes, white blood cells, neuro-peptides and etc.) to process a lot of denatured food. Food which had been largely stripped of its enzymic activity by cooking.

This would still be placing some food stress on my enzyme/immune system and this was what I sought to alleviate. I decided to switch to a mainly raw food diet. This was in line with my "juicing" habit mentioned earlier but it presented one major problem which I had to overcome — how to make quantities of raw food palatable?

Now I LIKE cooked food, it's what I'm used to. I like hot food and coming as I do from the north of a cold country I know the psychological value of "a good hot meal". So I wanted to continue these "comfort habits" whilst improving my diet. I began to think about hot food.

But just what is hot food, it's certainly not boiling food or roasting food or food that is at a temperature which will kill all its enzymes. No it's food that has been heated to the high temperatures involved in these processes in order to soften it, to make it easy to chew (but as we've seen not easier to digest) and then eaten as it cools.

Aeons ago we could only store our staple food surpluses by drying them and stacking them out of the way of the effects of light and damp, in granaries. When we came to use this stored staple, instead of soaking it in the light to bring it back to life we ground it up, mixed it with water and baked it into bread. Vegetables and fruits were either eaten in season, stored in "clamps" with considerable difficulty or boiled down to make jam or other concentrated forms of food. So the real reason that we began cooking in the first place was to make our staple foods easier to eat and to convert them into a more acceptable form when they could be stored, transported and distributed with ease.

Reasoning that we can now transport fresh foods around the world so as to be able to eat them out of season, and we can now store foods for long periods without the need for drying them, I realise that the main reason we began cooking food had been overcome. We no longer need to cook it to render it into chewable form, we can eat it fresh.

Looking at it this way I decided I could more or less pre-chew my raw food diet by grating, blending and liquidising it using all the electrical and mechanical apparatus in the kitchen.

That overcame the first hurdle but how to continue to enjoy hot food was still a problem.

I went back to my studies of water and looked at its energy curve. Water requires disproportionate amounts of energy to move it towards or away from the lowest point on its specific heat curve. To raise it from this temperature up to the temperature of boiling water at which the cellular structures of food can be ruptured and its texture made softer, requires a lot of energy input. This energy input costs a lot of money and as I no longer wanted to kill the food but simply to make it more easy to chew I had already solved that one and I didn't want to waste this money any more.

Like any other animals we don't actually like to eat hot food, what we really want is warm food. What we learned all those thousands of years ago when we began to eat cooked food, was that you have to cook it to make it soft enough to eat, but then you have to wait until its cooled down a bit before you can eat it. So what we have come to regard as hot food is really just food that has cooled down to close to our body temperature.

Moreover the water in food cooling down from boiling point towards the lowest point of its specific heat curve at plus 37 degrees Celsius, will be giving out oxygen rather than taking it in. Since the human body relies so heavily on oxygen I reason that food eaten at a temperature which is approaching the temperature of blood at plus 37.5 degrees Celsius will add to the body's oxygen supply and ergo its energy levels.

Simply put the body will not have to expend oxygen or heat energy to bring this food to a temperature at which the body can make the best use of it.

Now it's quite cheap and easy to get food up to body heat since that is the "home" temperature of water, and I found that one of the best and most palatable ways of doing this is to mix food which has been allowed to reach normal room temperature with a base (like a stock) which is hot (which has been boiled or otherwise cooked).

The mixing of the two or three masses has the effect of "diluting" the temperature of the "stock" and raising the temperature of the rest.

The other good method is to place the raw food preparation in a Bain Marie until it's warmed through.

In this way I was able to prepare and eat the "hot" food I had been used to since childhood, but now since it had not, in the main, been cooked, it retained all of its food value.

FLAVOURS

I found this to be a very good method of preparing food and one which introduced an enhanced range of flavours and textures into my life. Where previously I had been aware of and enjoyed the flavour of my food, now I began to enjoy it as it was in nature, before the flavour was reduced or substantially altered by cooking. All my food now tasted more strongly of its components and I had to experiment to find new permutations that I liked.

In this way I developed a whole new culinary art form and have detailed this in my cookery book "COOL COOKING" (the rejuvenation diet) obtainable from Sagax Publishing, 47 Haymill Close, Greenford, Middlesex UB6 8HL. Price £10.95 plus £2.00 postage and packing.

By the subtle use of spices and the correct combination of blended or hand-grated foods, with a cooked base, you can now enjoy an almost entirely natural diet full of living enzymes and nutritional value.

The hot and cold elements of these meals must be blended together in such a way, and in such quantities, as will ensure that the raw food component isn't heated to boiling point and so retains its enzymic activities. A bit of practice in this is needed but it soon brings success.

Likewise with flavours, you've got to relearn all the skills of cooking, but this time with the strength of the flavours of each of the ingredients much more in mind — then a whole new world of taste and enjoyment as well as health opens up to you.

TASTE

With this discovery a new dimension in life began. By this time I was already choosing fruit which was ripe and healthy for the juicing part of my diet and now I began to look for similar qualities in all my vegetables and food plants.

Rather than going on appearance I began to choose according to taste and this led me to another surprising and very beneficial discovery.

Locally produced organically grown food tastes far better than food grown on chemically treated soil!

We choose our food nowadays very largely on its appearance, how it looks, paying little attention to what it tastes like until we get it in the pot. This is a triumph of visuality over taste. We should first taste it and then choose, after all we're buying it to eat not to look at.

As my taste buds revived after years of abuse, I began to remember tastes and smells from my childhood, back in simpler days when salads were made from what my grandfather grew in his garden, on soil nourished by compost and manure.

I began to test different recipes on friends and noted a distinct preference amongst them for flavours of food which had been grown organically. More to the point I noticed that a switch to a diet made up entirely of organically grown uncooked foods slowed the ageing process. My hair stopped greying, my teeth stopped deteriorating, my eyesight improved and my virility increased! The illness which had started this odyssey disappeared completely and I resolved to continue the process of destressing and enhancing my life to ensure that I would live as long and as well as I was meant to, this time round!

### SHOOTS

Still concerned with the energy to be derived from different foods, I began to look at nature's growth patterns to see which periods in a plants life were the most energetic. Clearly when fruit or vegetables are coming into full ripeness there is a period of intense enzymic activity which culminates in the plant producing the most wonderfully complex sugars and enzymes to support its off-spring or to act as a store of food for its transition to the next year or next generation of its life.

This store is the most important source of food for all life on this planet but there is another point in a plant's life cycle where yet more energy is released into life, where yet more concentrated energy can be obtained.

This is at the point where new life springs from the old. Where a new shoot or sprout is formed.

Seeds and grains can lie dormant for thousands of years embedded in the dried out complex of stored food laid up for their use by their forebears. (Similarly dried fruit and vegetables can last quite a long time on the same basis). However once water is added to these seeds, the mechanism of the flow is re-established — electron transportation can take place and life can begin again.

Freshly sprouted seeds or grains are the most energetic life forms on the planet. They are the spark plugs of life, deriving huge amounts of energy from the newly activated stores of nutrients provided for them by the previous generation and literally sparkling with life when viewed on kirlian photographs.

At no other time in a plant's life is so much energy made available in its metabolism and this energy — because of its huge enzymic activity is readily available to humans.

With this discovery I was able to begin to add bulk to my diet and have more to chew on again. I sprouted trays of seeds and mixed the resultant harvest into my food as well as developing a wide range of salads by mixing various sprouts together. I also applied the same principle of (adding fresh water) to supplies of dried nuts and this provided me with a much more satisfying and easy to digest supply of protein than I had previously been able to get from dried nuts. They are much easier and better to eat when soaked.

I go into this whole process of sprouting different grains and seeds in my book "Cool Cooking" but you can easily arrive at conclusions which will suit you equally well by experimenting in your own kitchen.

There is no secret to this, primitive tribes and also people in advanced civilisations to this day derive enormous benefit in their diet from eating sprouting shoots and these seared (or slightly singed) in a Wok make a wonderfully palatable yet still largely uncooked source of highly energetic food.

### MONEY

The upshot of these discoveries was that I began not only to be a lot more healthy and vigorous, but I also had a lot more money to spare at the end of each month. The reason for this was that I now use very little fuel energy to cook food. (Admittedly it costs money to juice and blend raw food but not nearly as much as it costs to cook it!) I now buy less of all the food stuffs I eat. (Once again the organic foods I eat are more expensive than the visually attractive rubbish I used to buy, but they are more energy rich and I use less of them, so it balances out). I now buy quantities of dried grains and seeds very cheaply for sprouting. These supply a large component of my diet because they are so energy-rich once I have sprouted them.

Storage is no problem because most of the seeds I buy are naturally dried so refrigeration is less important than it used to be. Also raw foods keep a lot longer and better than cooked foods because their cellular structure remains intact and they do not begin to rot down so readily.

I am richer and healthier for these rather obvious discoveries and the change of diet has taught me a great deal in the way of useful skills. I have become involved in life, with life, again. Less self-obsessed.

This notion of becoming less self-obsessed is very useful when you're ill since it helps you to focus your mind on something else other than your illness and represents the beginning of renewed mental health as we will see later.

### AIR

Living in the last phase of an industrial society it is difficult to breathe fresh air, particularly in cities, because of all the pollutants dumped into it. From my researches into air ionisation it had become obvious that a good supply of fresh "living" air, that is to say air which has a high degree of electronic activity associated with and provided by living systems, was essential to a healthy energy-rich existence.

It's relatively easy to filter the bulk of particulates and bacteria out of air but to do so is a very expensive business and at the end of it you finish up with denatured air, which as we've seen in Chapter Three, is very bad for your health.

The only natural sources of healthy air are provided, in the cities, by parks, gardens, recreation grounds and playing fields. Here you can breathe air which is provided with a healthy component of electronic activity by the life systems of the vegetation. Going for long walks in these areas or better still in forested areas in the country provides a much needed boost to vitality.

I found that these walks were even more beneficial if taken during or just after a rain shower as then the air is particularly active being full of the electrical charges created by falling water droplets. Falling water droplets create tiny dipol charges which renew the energy lattice of the air by imparting negative charges (electrons) to air molecules.

This is why sitting by a fountain or waterfall is so good for health and so calming, fountains and waterfalls release negative ions into the air. These suffuse the body with energy via the lungs and the meridians so reducing the seratonin content of the blood which has a calming yet invigorating effect on the whole brain-body system, as we've seen.

Recognising this effect I also began to take regular showers in preference to baths. Showers, particularly cool or cold ones are invigorating partly because the cold water stimulates the blood flow to the surface of the skin but also because they generate substantial quantities of negatively charged air ions. However there is a limited number of showers you want to take in a day and I wanted to find other ways, additional ways, to reduce the stress placed on my system by polluted, denatured, air.

My sprout growing programme was already well under way and by their nature growing plants, particularly sprouts, emits streams of electrons from their tips into the air. To supplement these I decided to get an air ioniser of the type described in Chapter Three.

Most of the air ionisers on the market are cheap rubbish stemming from the fact that there was a boom in air ioniser production in the sixties and seventies. This boom stemmed from the publicity given to the initial discoveries of the beneficial effects of air ionisation. But this publicity was basically high-jacked by crude commercial interests who know very little about the subject and simply sought to make the maximum profit from it. Accordingly exaggerated claims were made then for air ionisation and in the end things got so out of hand that the FDA in the USA quite rightly decided to ban all advertising which made medical claims for ionisers. This ban was followed by a similar one in the UK and so greed just about killed off a promising branch of scientific research.

In many ways the advertising ban was a bit like throwing the baby out with the bath water as it put paid to several companies who were motivated by the good of their customers' health in addition to making a profit. But some of the people involved in the early research and who were involved in those companies are still around and still able to make really effective kit given the opportunity to do so. (Oh, the snake oil and bullshit people are still there too, but they, like Pifco and Dezak etc., have found a very ready market for low-grade ionisers in catalogues and pharmacy chain stores.) I took time to look at the whole ioniser situation and then commission a small company with an excellent research and development background in ionisation to make a device to my own specifications. This device is basically an industrial, fan-driven, electron generator with an unique function. It blows out a plume of biologically available electrons into the air of my house. These create a power lattice in the air which builds, over a period of time, into a very healthy air environment.

The first effects are the precipitation of all dust particulates from the air and as I live in London this means that all the diesel particulates plate-out on to the walls and floor, and not on to my lungs.

Next, all my plants began to grow more vigorously and put out foilage more actively.

Cross-infection is reduced as the air-borne bacteria and virus are wiped out, and for the first time in years I no longer caught the vigorous colds my children brought home from school. Nor did they reinfect each other any more.

My beloved younger son Thomas is hyperactive and slowly but surely as the lattice/"fresh living air" effect of the "Progenitor" built up, we noticed that he calmed down a bit. This is probably due to the seratonin reduction effect that a negatively charged atmosphere causes.

Finally my sleep patterns improved and I was able to sleep more deeply and get better rest than I had for years.

## REAL AEROBIC EXERCISE

In order to increase my vitality and charge myself up to full living vigour, I began to exercise each day, directly in the plume of air put out by the "Progenitor". I found that this enabled me to breathe more deeply and more slowly when exercising, allowing for a more sustained output of energy during my exercises.

In the course of my studies I have come across examples of people who lived in the unpolluted pre-industrial environment of our ancestors, and were able to perform prodigious feats of endurance. I imagine that I've gone some way toward recreating the environment they lived in when I exercise in front of my own personal vast store of natural living bacteria-free air.[*]

Certainly an enhanced "living air" atmosphere helped speed up my recovery and helps me stay vigorously healthy in today's sick environment.

Finally on the subject of the Progenitor:

Several years ago I suffered a very bad head injury which was not treated at the time. Subsequently I was diagnosed as having a thinning bone in my neck. This often bears down on a nerve and causes pain in my left shoulder.

More recently, when I had unthinkingly placed myself in a situation that I should have avoided, I had an accident when I tripped over a cable and fell banging my head on the floor and breaking two ribs. This seems to have triggered off or set up a fault in my left side functioning the result of which is that I keep having accidents where I hit things with my left arm or hand when I'm walking past them. My left side co-ordination is a bit out.

The result of this is a number of minor injuries to my left hand — and these heal faster in the "plume" of the Progenitor than when I am away from it.

[*] For bactericide effect see Product Index

From this it would seem that not only are air-borne electrons able to disinfect air but they also actively promote healing.

This is probably a function of the ability of the body to transport electrons throughout its structure via the lungs and the meridians. But it may also be a direct effect of an electron-enriched atmosphere on the biological reactions taking place on the surface of the skin.

Certainly all of our complexions have been improved since I began using the progenitor.

# CHAPTER TEN

## *CONCLUSION*

### WATER

In Chapter Eight under the heading "Living Energies" I wrote:

> "The vortices and their dynamics which are associated with pathcurve forms intimately relate to the water which forms up to 90 per cent of our structures, also to the organic processes taking place inside any living organism".

I went on to say that:

> "They relate the life forces to physical substance through the medium of form acting upon water and imprinting on its micro-structures".

What I'm driving at here is that pathcurve forms set up force fields around themselves and these force fields imprint themselves particularly and peculiarly on water. They structure water.

From the very beginning life on this planet formed out of a cooperation between the properties of life forces flowing through structures in water and it is very clear from my research that the one cannot exist without the other (on this planet in any event).

This process of the transfer of flow from the metaphysical to the physical is basic to life and is facilitated and arbitrated by water.

Thus water is the most important substance to life on this planet and it was to the water we drink that I next turn my attention in my quest for full good health.

### HEALTHY WATER

Water is the carrier substance, the bearer of life on earth, and as such it is very important to full good health to drink "healthy" water.

At first the idea of healthy water may seem a bit odd especially since the current view of water holds that it is simply $H_2O$, a simple liquid. However as we saw in Chapter Five, water is the most complex and interesting of substances and forms a crucial part of our diet, as well as a vital component in our lives.

The fact that water can dissolve substances out of our bodies as well as acting as the bearer of substances going into our structures is obviously the most relevant physical attribute of water to our daily lives. But the fact that it can also transport information in and out of our bodies is perhaps yet more important when we're looking at the subtle forces which set up the precursor conditions for good or ill-health.

In my quest for a stress free life I decided to first deal with the physical aspects of water.

### WATER-BORNE DISEASES

In the recent past we've suffered badly from water-borne diseases such as cholera and typhoid and as part of a two-pronged attack on these we began to chlorinate our drinking water to kill off all the pathogenic bacteria.

We'd arrived at a state of getting such diseases as cholera and typhoid largely because we had begun to clump together in large towns and cities which were (a) poorly supplied with fresh uncontaminated drinking water and (b) had little or no sewage disposal except a drain running down the middle of each street.

Under these circumstances it's hardly surprising that there were regular outbreaks of these horrible diseases and the main prong of the attack in eradicating these was the provision and development (in Victorian times) of an efficient sewage disposal system.

Once sewage and all the other rat infested garbage and filth began to be disposed of elsewhere than in the streets. Once it was taken away and dealt with thoroughly then the incidence of these diseases fell off, yet it was still considered necessary to filter and chlorinate our water supplies to ward off any accidental infestation.

The purification and transportation of water are now one

of our major industries and yet despite the scale of operation of these industries they still operate on the crudest of lines when it comes to the actual treatment of the water itself.

This is unfortunate because there are available nowadays brilliantly simple (as most complex concepts usually turn out to be in practice) methods of treating and transporting water which will purify it and clean it in the process of its transportation. (If anybody reading this would like to know more about these methods please drop me a line and I will be pleased to enlighten you).

Turning back now to chlorination, chlorination and in some instances fluoridation, sterilise water to try to remove all micro-organisms and pathogenic bacteria. In its function as a water steriliser or disinfectant, chlorine eradicates all types of bacteria, beneficial and harmful alike, so what arrives at the tap or faucet for our use, while free of every possible organism, has been sterilised to death.

Healthy water like healthy food should contain a balance of naturally occurring bacteria and micro-organisms. This is the kind of water we evolved with in our natural state and it is normal and healthy for us to drink fresh pure spring water with a wide range of minerals dissolved in it (and a wide range of bacteria present). Our immune systems are designed to deal with any pathogens very effectively but they are not designed to deal with disinfectants!

When we drink water with chlorine dissolved in it we are taking into our bodies a poisonous gas (chlorine), which kills all bacteria and micro-organisms. As we've seen earlier the cells of our bodies are micro-organisms, our gut is full of beneficial bacteria and micro-organisms. Our entire immune system is made up almost in its entirety of beneficial micro-organisms.

In drinking chlorinated water therefore we are actually sterilising our blood, thereby weakening our immune system and setting up in our bodies the conditions in which disease can flourish.

By the time it gets to us chlorinated water isn't a particularly strong disinfectant but it's a very persistent one and in the West we drink it every day of our lives. In doing so we steadily and eventually impair our immune systems to such a degree that they are no longer able to eject virus, germs and cancer cells.

## IMPURITIES

Modern supplies of treated water come into contact with a wide range of chemicals, plastics, metals and other organic and inorganic substances which are usually removed before the water reaches our homes. However the process of removing these impurities does not remove their imprint from the clathrate micro-structures of water. Thus when this water arrives in our homes for us to drink there are bound up in its structures the imprint or "memory" of these substances which can include of course lead or cadmium or PCB's etc. These killer poisons have unique resonant "signatures" and these signatures are passed into the water in our body for our immune system to deal with. Similarly modern water supplies come into contact with or are exposed to powerful electromagnetic fields such as are generated by high-tension three-phase pylons or micro-wave antenna etc.

The metal pipes that carry a substantial proportion of our water supply can be shown to be conducting not only the fluctuating background geomagnetic flow of current, but also many more localised currents such as the above, that they pick up as they pass in the vicinity of these artificial power sources.

## THE WRONG SPIN

The bulk of these currents as well as the bulk of broadcast power in the form of micro-waves, radio-waves, radar etc., is of an artificially generated nature. It is therefore capable of imparting the wrong spin to water. Or setting up the anti-clockwise vortex effect of magnetism. As we saw earlier in the chapter dealing with water vortices these artificially generated vortices do not occur in nature and are the products of an artificially generated electromagnetic field.

Those vortices which occur naturally in the body have a clockwise spin, therefore when we drink tap water or any other water not occurring in natural springs or deep wells, then there is a strong possibility that we are importing into our bodies a substance which places a heavy stress on our systems. It does so because our bodies have to re-orientate it or cancel out its effects before this water can be normalised and property integrated into our systems.

This costs energy and represents a continual challenge to our immune systems at a very basic sometimes sub-molecular level.

### DISSOLVED MINERALS

Finally concerning the mineral and oxygen content of our drinking water:

Naturally occurring ground water which issues to the surface in springs has a wide range of minerals dissolved into it from the rocks that have passed through during its time underground. It invariably reaches the surface at a temperature of around plus 4 degrees Celsius or in other words at or close to its anomaly point, at which point, as we saw earlier, it is most dense and energetic.

When it reaches the surface in this form it is almost totally lacking in dissolved oxygen which it proceeds to absorb at a quite prodigious rate. It thereby increases its volume substantially in its first few metres of flow at the surface and, as its temperature rises, begins to add to its mineral content by absorbing something of what it comes into contact with.

Spring water splashing down a mountain and through the shade of its accompanying vegetation contains the natural, healthy, energetic components that we evolved to drink and this balanced oxygen and mineral content is mediated by its temperature as we shall see.

### RIPE WATER

I decided to think biologically and set up a system which would come as close as possible to replicating nature and its production of ripe water. That is to say water which contains the right, most biologically useful, mix of minerals and oxygen. But water without the poisonous influences of chlorine, metallic/chemical imprints or electromagnetic field effects. I went to work on my homes main water supply.

### REMOVING ELECTROMAGNETIC POLLUTION FROM WATER

To do this I bought and fitted a device which, using a coil of wire wrapped round the rising main. This scrambles all the electromagnetic signals and poison signals bound in the micro-structures (clathrates) of the water coming into my home. Not only did this randomise the signals in the clathrate structures (which was what I was trying to do) but it also had the beneficial side-effect of restructuring the dissolved limestone content in the water which made it softer and easier to wash with. These devices are quite common and I actually bought a Krystal unit from Carefree in the United Kingdom. Similar products supplied by Water King are equally as good for this purpose (and please see the Appendices of this book for the addresses of various suppliers).

In this way I succeeded in removing all the coherent or characteristic patterns and frequencies from the water coming into my house and achieved electromagnetically cleaned water with a random pattern which I could then begin to structure in the way I wanted.

### REMOVING CHEMICAL POLLUTION FROM WATER

The next phase was to remove all the gross chemical and bacteriological impurities if any, from the main supply. I reasoned that there probably wouldn't be many bacteria present owing to the excessive chlorination of our supply, but I noticed marked fluctuations in the levels of chlorine in the tap water over a period of time and was suspicious of its quality. This especially after a couple of hot summers had shown how vulnerable this could be.

Moreover I wanted to pass the water through a reverse osmosis filter after it had been electromagnetically randomised so as to take out as much chlorine as possible.

I bought and fitted a rather expensive miniature reverse osmosis water filtering which allegedly only allows molecules of pure water to pass through the membrane. In sequence after this I fitted another more simple device containing activated carbon granules in silver as a second/third stage in my water treatment process. I was content that at the end of this effort I was at least getting water that was relatively clean and had a good chance of not containing many of the quite virulent manmade toxins that are now seeping into our water supplies.

All this effort made the water taste slightly better and I now wanted to begin to treat my drinking water in such a way as would help it towards the characteristics I most needed.

### LEFT-HAND RIGHT-HAND

I particularly wanted to overcome and eradicate those left spinning vortices in water which puts such a strain on living systems. This is very important from the point of view of full health because it is these structures which (a) represent a physical challenge on the micro-structure level insofar as they deform the flow of the body's energy requiring constant correction and thus energy use in the body, and (b) as we've seen at the beginning of this chapter vortices have the effect of imprinting vibrations of other substances on the water which they come to inhabit. Thus left spinning vortices are the main culprits in the transfer of electromagnetic "impurities" to water in the body as well as being the main culprit of the transfer of "poison memory" vibrations into the clathrate structures of the body.

To finally eradicate any memory of these inappropriate vortices I bought a spiraliser. These devices available in the UK from Aquarian Angel Services Limited (see address in Appendix) are made up of a funnel which contains a tin-plated copper spiral. This spiral gives a right hand spin to all liquids poured through the funnel and dramatically improves their taste, aroma and wholesomeness. Basically it does this by making them much easier for our bodies to use since they're spinning in the same direction as all of the vortices throughout our body thus causing no difference patterns in collision with these but cooperating with them and adding energy into our systems.

Much earlier in this book I mentioned the different chiral states of molecules (ie their left- or right-handedness) as having different smells and tastes, and this improvement in the taste of liquids passed through a spiraliser is simply an example on a gross scale of the principle of "handedness" in action.

Using this three stage process of electromagnetically scrambling, physically filtering and spiralling our drinking water I was now getting close to the supply I wanted. However reasoning that water needed to absorb both oxygen, some minerals and reach a stable temperature I decided to go yet further in the water treatment process.

Looking at how nature stores valuable fluids I noticed that the egg-shape is her preferred form of vessel. Going back over the work on pathcurves and pathcurve structures, I perceived that there was an opportunity here to bring or encourage the subtle forces used by nature in and around these structures, to work on my drinking water.

I decided to store water for several days before using it in an egg-shaped vessel where it could benefit from the flow of energy around these shapes.

### AMPHORA

Beginning to search for a supply of these vessels I came on another discovery which confirmed my findings:

All ancient civilisations used these shapes in which to store water, wine and oil.

The Egyptians, Greeks, Sumarians, Hitites, Romans, Japanese (Jyomoun-doki water storage jars) and a host of other ancient and very durable civilisations used the amphora for storing grain and liquids! They used to store almost everything valuable that had a fluid nature in these or in "Ali baba" jars which have a similar internal shape.

Now amphora are logically a very poor shape for compact and efficient storage. They come down to a point and are fairly slender. They are difficult to stack and give the appearance of being quite fragile. Worst of all they take up a lot of space. So why did all of the ancient civilisations use them almost exclusively for the long-term storage of valuable fluids?

The answer is simple:

These containers both encourage and allow the subtle flows of beneficial energy through their structures. They contain no stagnant zones, no right-handed corners (that can inhibit flowing movement and provide a suitable environment for pathogenic bacteria to breed). Rather they are formed of spiral curves where healthy flowing life-giving movement can take place.

By placing these earthenware vessels in shaded areas, exposed to moving air, changes of temperature are induced. These changes in temperature induce all movements in gases and liquids so that what is stored in an amphora (a path curve vessel) is subject to gentle spiralling movements exemplified by heat exchange and is therefore able to become more vital and better balanced.

NATURE'S COOLERS

Amphora are a bit hard to come by in Northern Europe and so I began to experiment with different materials to see if I could get the same effect. I found that natural stone or wooden barrels did the job very well but for ease of use and aesthetic reasons I finally tracked down a supply of unglazed amphora. The unglazed aspect of terracotta was very important to me because I wanted to allow my drinking water to cool naturally. Because its porous terracotta is particularly well suited to water storage since it enables a very small percentage of the contents of the vessel to evaporate through the vessel walls. Evaporation allows for cooling and therefore I reason that by placing my amphora in a shaded position with a good air flow the water stored in them would cool down steadily and stabilise somewhere near its anomaly point. Its state of highest energy or health.

I experimented with this and it worked so I now had a system which cleaned and purified my drinking water, plus a system which cooled it and gave it the correct polarity. All that remained was to provide a natural blend of minerals for it to absorb.

ROCK MEAL

As we saw at the beginning of Chapter One all life began on

earth with a combination of a coming together of minerals dissolved from rocks and energy flows derived from movements, in the medium of water. I reasoned that water at its highest energy point would normally dissolve a complex of minerals in such proportions as are beneficial to life and I went in search of collaboration of this.

Living in the high Himalayas of northern Pakistan, the Hunza are one of the most healthy people on earth with average life expectancies between 130 and 140 years. Their fields are watered by cold glacier melt water which is rich in trace elements which have been ground from the rocks over which the glacier has passed.

Their fields are therefore constantly fertilised with a broad spectrum of minerals. These fields not only maintain a high level of productivity but the produce itself is vibrantly healthy and disease free.

Clearly the naturally occurring mineral complex dissolved in the water close to its anomaly point was what was in action here and I elected to provide my drinking water with what it obviously needed to make its contribution to my full health.

I went to a local quarry which is in the business of crushing rock for road building, and bought a bag of crusher dust which is basically finely crushed gravel or basalt. I then got a small bag made of rot-proof fibre (artificial fibre), filled this with rock dust and suspended it in my water storage jars.

In order to allow the water to "work" in the jars and absorb the optimum amount of minerals I left it standing for three days. At the end of this time I used the resultant "ripe" water for two weeks to irrigate my sprouting trays.

The results were dramatic, my sprouts now grew at approximately twice their previous rate, achieving a water uptake and weight which was remarkable. Moreover they were vigorous and vital clearly thriving on this new regime.

I took this to be all the proof I needed to begin using the "ripe" water myself and since I had been eating the sprouts watered by it for several days, I ran no extra risk from doing so.

The results have been quite significant, for a start everything now tastes much better. Although it's not a word usually used to describe taste I would say that all my drinks taste much "softer". They also have a lot more flavour. The main effects however have been in my gross health. I felt less tired and more vital on this regime. My appetite is better and I feel more optimistic. Clearly I am now getting something positive from my drinking water and have eradicated much of the stress that I previously had to deal with from this source.

### SINGING SAND

For more than a century scientists have known that sand can occasionally make loud booming noises or small squeaks, but until recently it was not known what caused this effect. The results of a team working on this were published in *Nature* magazine in March '97 and reported in *New Scientist* magazine in the same month.

The team which comprised chemist Douglas Goldsak of Laurentian University plus Marcel Leech and Cindi Kilkeny discovered that the singing sands have a sparkling dust-free surface. Infra-red spectroscopy showed this to be partly composed of water and partly of dissolved silica (which comes from finally crushed sand redeposited on the surface of sand grains which had absorbed water). This silica and water mix forms a gel and this sticky coating allows the sand grains to adhere together. This causes the whole sandune to behave like a giant tuning fork and the frequency of the tone emitted seems to depend on the size of the sand grains involved.

That silica and water can bond together and resonate as a structure is all important to the next step in the destressing process:

### PROTECTING YOURSELF FROM ELECTROMAGNETIC FIELD EFFECTS

Vibrating information patterns in water aren't very stable, they can be degraded by freezing, radioactivity, bright sunlight and by exposure to electromagnetic fields.

This is like saying that whilst water has a memory it doesn't have a very good one! However the memory can be fixed, it can be set into a relatively permanent form by mixing it with silica. Silica grains, like everything else in nature, are usually covered by a very thin film of water. If this water on the silica grains is imprinted with vibrating patterns then these become very stable and withstand strong electromagnetic fields without the pattern becoming degraded.

Water has an affinity for silica similar to its affinity for carbon and its often been thought that if life hadn't evolved on this planet with a carbon base then it would have evolved with a silicon base because of this.

### COPPER WIRE

It's usual to think as most things around the house as being dry, and on a gross level that's true. However on a microscopic level just about everything at room temperature is covered by a very thin film of water. This water isn't liquid in the sense that it will run about the place but is a film stuck to the surface of everything.

All electrical conductors that we use are metal and most of them are copper. Copper is composed of myriad tiny crystals and on the outer surface of the crystals of copper wire is a thin film of water.

In the normal course of events when a current is passed along the wire it will set up a magnetic field at right angles to the flow of current.

This magnetic field will generate a series of vortices along the length of the wire through the vibrations induced in the water. These vortices will have an anti-clockwise rotation and extend well above and below the wire. These are the effects to be guarded against in the home or any living or working environment since it is these vortices having the wrong spin which "disturb" the water in our bodies damaging or degrading its clockwise life-system spin (vortex form).

Let me recapitulate. As we've seen water has a micro-structure into which vibrational patterns can be fixed/imprinted. These micro-structures aren't all the same and their properties vary but certain of these have properties that distinguish them from all the others when they are imprinted onto silica powder. They can form an energy vortex (even in the absence of a specific pathcurve form).

In the case of silica the form is actually in the water microstructure itself. And so a sufficient quantity of silica made into a compact "brick" will generate a strong vortex. This vortex can be further amplified by making a triangular arrangement of three such piles and the result is physically very simple but very complex at a molecular level.

This arrangement generates a very strong vortex moving vertically downwards in a clockwise direction. As it passes through the silica it picks up the vibrational information patterned from the water film on the silica. If a metallic wire is then placed into this vortex, the water on the surface of the wire is set vibrating with the frequencies in the vortex. This can then propagate through the water on the surface of the wire because this water is in intimate contact with the crystal structure of the copper. In this way vibrations that originate in the water on the silica can be spread down a wire for a distance of at least fifty metres.

The vibration generated in the water film on the wire in this way is strong enough to prevent any other vibration being set up by any magnetic fields around the wire. So in the wires carrying electricity, which means that it would be generating magnetism, this magnetism is not able to create the disturbance in the water that it would otherwise make.

This system completely blocks the anti-clockwise vortex effect of the artificially generated magnetism!

THE SOLUTION

When this wire is connected to the wiring system of a house the vibrating effect caused by the brick vortex device is transmitted to all the wiring and into every piece of electrical apparatus that it is connected to. In this way the negative effect of any magnetic field is prevented at source, that is to say inside the machines and the wiring itself, and prevented from doing damage to living systems in its area.

The magnetic field generated by the flow of electricity is not of course affected but the situation is dramatically changed in the water which this magnetic field comes into contact with.

In any building there is usually a lot of wire hidden away under floors, across ceilings in walls and so forth so that we live in what are actually very complex cages of copper wire. When the whole of such a system of wires is set vibrating from a silica source, then the effect spreads out into the space within and any magnetic fields have no effect on any water in this space. In other words, it builds a bio-dynamic field the size of the building.

This is quite a complex process but the end result is very simple. If a simple vortex generator is plugged into the mains wiring then a bio-dynamic field is set up which blocks the harmful effect that any magnetic field set up by the flow of electricity would otherwise have on water.

On discovering this I immediately bought one of these vortex units and plugged it in. To my delight it worked extremely well and it transpires that the vortex unit is not only able to deal with disturbances whose source is from within the building but also with disturbances from external sources, those which come up from the ground or in through the walls. Clearly then this unit is able to generate a bio-dynamic field of adequate strength to protect living systems from the harmful effects of electromagnetic fields whatever their source.

In use it does not of course change either the electric or magnetic fields in the area. These are still present and still measurable. What it does is it changes the impact that the electromagnetic fields have on water.

Using this device on a permanent basis now I have found that I sleep much better now that I am free from electrical or geopathic stress. Also several irritating harmonics that were coming from various electrical apparatus around the house have died away making the overall environment a lot more healthy.

Vortex units can be obtained from Sagax Publishing. See Appendices.

## EXORCISING STRESS

It's very unusual for anyone to get cancer in the arms or legs or in the bones or muscles. It's not unheard of but it's rare. This is due to the fact that these parts of the body are mobile and are able to transmit stress into movement. They react to stress by moving and, by undertaking this mechanical function, they transform irritation into activity.

Broadly speaking organs that are able to do this, to transfer energy into activity, are unlikely to suffer from the hyper-stress which can cause cancer. Those organs which cannot do this, like all of the fixed soft tissue organs in the body, often do.

So clearly exercise and "work" are very useful in eliminating stress from the body and it is to the type of exercise we should look in the process of helping ourselves.

## EMOTIONAL STRESS

Broadly speaking the mind, as we've seen, works on three levels. The unconscious, which is part of the vast mind of the Universal Creative Intelligence. The subconscious, which is the huge engine of our personalities and the conscious which is the focus of the neo-cortex.

When the conscious perceives an event or series of events as being contrary to its way of looking at things, that is to say opposed to or at odds with its dominant mental state then it responds to this by being irritated. This irritation is amplified on the emotional level (the emotions being the way the subconscious responds to events) and this combination of conscious and subconscious unease results in a complex of neuro-hormones being secreted into the bloodstream which cause the body to respond in a certain way.

This response is one which reduces the efficiency of the immune system (which in this context can be looked upon as a circulating nervous system), which in turn diminishes the flow of life forces through the body by setting up resistances or a resistance to its smooth passage.

As we saw earlier the smooth passage of the life-force is fundamental to the regular and optimum creation of the correct or optimum proportion of red and white blood cells in the body. Thus once a negative feedback loop is established it becomes very difficult to break.

### DOMINANT MENTAL STATE

The dominant mental state of your mind is your method of looking at things. It represents the "filter" of emotions, attitudes and anxieties which are your habitual response to stimuli and it dictates your response.

Therefore if you have become ill using your present dominant mental attitude it's axiomatic that you must change it in order to get better. In turn this will change your responses and will thus change the rate and proportion of the secretion of neuro-hormones into your blood stream which mediate the flow of the life-force through you.

### HOW TO CHANGE YOUR DOMINANT MENTAL ATTITUDE

Stress in the body usually involves emotions. An upset can make us tense and nervous, almost all the emotional reactions cause us to tighten our stomach muscles and our breathing becomes shallow and rapid, or difficult and laboured when we feel threatened. These stresses accumulate in the stomach and lungs, in the shoulders or the spine, and unless we discharge them they can make us ill.

Just as we've seen that the dominant mental attitude amplified through the emotions is what can cause us to be ill, now we're going to turn that on its head, and observe how we can set up the conditions whereby we can change our dominant mental attitude by the simple process of working backwards from our emotions. That is to say by changing our emotions so as to ultimately change our mind-set (the way we look at things).

The best way to guard against the effects of stress is to become involved in some regular form of exercise by which this stress is dissipated into a constructive activity. When I first became ill I bought an exercise machine, one which purports to exercise every muscle set in the body, and I began to use this regularly every morning.

Apart from being physically challenging at first I found this activity extremely boring until I hit upon a device by which I could control my mental activity and still my runaway thoughts.

I taught myself to meditate, and to do so I began to focus my attention by learning to fix my mind on the air passing my nostrils. This was very difficult to do at first but with practice I was able to go into this activity at will, and slowly but surely I gained control of my thoughts. Each time my mind began to wander I would bring it back to what I wanted it to do, and as the endless chatter began again each time, I would halt it and bring my mind back to the air passing the tip of my nose.

Now this may seem an utterly pointless exercise, but think a minute - if you've got your attention fixed on something you can't become preoccupied or involved in something else. The focus of your mind is simply incapable of concentrating on two things at once. You can't do it! So when you focus hard on one thing ALL YOUR EMOTIONAL ACTIVITY CALMS DOWN! You become calm inside, your glandular balance rights itself and your body can then begin to clear up the toxic states created by the secretion of complexes of hormones in response to earlier powerful or irritating emotions.

If whilst you are in this mental state your body is working on some rhythmic physical function, then you will be supplying it with adequate oxygen and energy flows for it to flex all of its systems and allow the trapped energy to discharge into motion — movement.

If you perform such an exercise each morning you will eventually become very strong and healthy and your self-esteem will grow. There is no need to overdo it but you must perform a regular fairly challenging exercise for a set time each day if you want to become really fit and well (both physically and mentally).

Another very good exercise for this purpose is walking. As you walk you can very easily calm your mind and fix your attention onto something on the horizon so as to exclude the mental chatter. Also walking is very good for your circulation, since every time you put your foot down you compress the capillaries under your foot which causes the blood to shoot up the veins in your legs, thus helping it on its way back to the lungs and heart. This is natures foot pump in action.

On the subject of walking however, it should be noted that a short walk will not de stress or exercise you, you need to walk at least three miles a day, regularly, in order to get the full benefit of this activity.

Finally on the subject of low stress regular exercise:

Both long distance swimming and rowing are extremely good for you since they and similar exercises provide the rhythmic release needed each day, but the list more or less stops there, because of the need to be wide awake and aware of your surroundings during most other sporting activities.

### ANGER

Clearly, I'm talking here of emotions being susceptible to amelioration by exercise and it would be unwise to leave this section without dealing with an extremely damaging emotion.

Violence is the outcome of anger, if the violence has no way of venting it will turn inward in time and hurt you. This energy has to go somewhere and so to avoid it going into you and accumulating in your organs as stress, when you become furiously angry you should go and chop wood, dig the garden, go somewhere private and rant and rave for a couple of minutes, hit a punch bag, jump on a trampoline, quickly do a bungy jump or a parachute jump, dive in a pool or run somewhere as fast as you can — above all else find a way to discharge your anger so that it can't hurt you or anyone else.

### GROWING

Once I learned how to discharge stress effectively through exercise and moving meditation I then reasoned that a complete change in the way I was living was essential to bring me back to optimum good health. Accordingly I began to do the things that I really enjoy doing and did a lot less of the things that had put stress on me in the first place. I also looked for activities which would involve me more with life and help me to see things in perspective, or I should say in a different perspective, so that they would not upset me so much.

I realised that it's very difficult to hold on to stress if you're involved with growing living things. For example gardening is a wonderful calming pursuit in which the gardener cultivates the earth and, in turn, the earth cultivates the gardener.

Several research projects are on record where prisons have been involved in trying to help their more violent and difficult in-mates by encouraging them to cultivate allotments of land. In every case even the most violent psychopaths have calmed down and taken an interest in this activity to the point where most have become substantially rehabilitated and able to be released.

Involvement with living creatures which depend on you for their support and healthy development brings out the best in everyone and helps each of us to redefine and reassess our role in relation to life so as to take a more balanced healthy direction.

### YOUR GROWTH

Most people, or at least a substantial majority of people, who get cancer have had an appalling shock in their lives, like the loss of a loved one, or the loss of the main role in their lives, which they found so supportive of their self-view.

Others in this category have suffered some severe disappointment or setback which has depressed them badly. Yet others have had a severe physical blow which has left them badly shaken.

In each of these cases the individual's world view and self-view has been sorely challenged and when this happens a person's moods become melancholy, they lose confidence and begin to doubt their purpose. This state of mind suppresses the immune system and they become susceptible to stress. As this stress builds up they internalise it, wishing to keep up appearances, until it breaks out in severe illness which then depresses them even further. This becomes a negative feedback loop.

This kind of thing which usually comes along in late middle age is very common, as I've said, and it's very difficult to get over. It requires great courage and strength of character to effect the necessary changes but, if by this stage you've been following the thinking in this book you'll have begun to change already and you'll now know that you have what it takes to change your life.

### CHANGE

From talking to many people who have made themselves ill by living unhealthy lives a remarkable fact has emerged:

Most people want to get better so that they can go back to their old ways and return to their old life-style!

This you cannot do! Your old life is what made you ill in the first place and if you go back to living that way, it will kill you!

You must now change your life, learn to live another way, become someone different. If you do not effect deep down changes in the way you've been living then you will not get better, or if you do you will not stay better for long.

Let's look at this another way:

> If you've become ill with dread disease then the fiat of ill-health has gone out against you, against the being you are. Nature has decided that it no longer has a use for you (at least not in your present form). You are being told in no uncertain terms that despite whatever you may feel or think, the greater whole, the Universal Creative Intelligence, has decided that it can no longer learn from your existence in its present form.

Clean living, medical science and a strong will may prolong your life for a while but unless you consciously decide to change direction you're going to live a poor shadow of what you were before.

### NEW DIRECTIONS

To take a new direction in life is perhaps the most difficult thing you will ever have to do because it involves looking hard at the person you've become, the personality you feel safe and secure within, and consciously deciding to let go of this carapace and begin to grow again.

The purpose of life is growth, creativity and learning. By serving this purpose you can grow again, become healthy and useful, and go once again into the flow of creation.

Looking back over my life when I became ill, I realised that I had come to a turning point, I had reached a point where I either had to learn and develop a new purpose, or die. I decided at that time to learn as much as I could about the illness that had brought me to the end of that life and use that information to write this book so as to help other people to restart their lives and grow to full good health again.

REPROGRAMMING

Realising that the most difficult part of this regime is changing a person's dominant mental attitude I developed a whole-brain learning technique which helped me to do this. Initially my purpose in working on this method, which is called the Flow programme, was that, like most people, I get lazy and forgetful. I begin everything with a spate of good intentions but as time goes by my good intentions go by the board and I tend to slide back into old and "comfortable" ways.

This sort of thing is no good at all if you're facing the enormous challenge of dread disease and so I wrote out and recorded on cassette tape a number of scripts which I use to remind myself each day of my new direction.*

The whole point of the Flow programme is to teach and show you the listener, how to replace negative, worn out old

---

\* If you think this kind of programme might be supportive or helpful in your efforts then you can buy it through my publishers Sagax Publishing, 47 Haymill Close, Greenford, Middlesex UB6 8HL at £75 a set of tapes. These come to you in a beautiful little wooden box of five tapes and this programme is designed to run for a month at a rate of one lesson per day, each lesson lasting about 15 minutes. As I said the whole point of this exercise is to help you to stay on course and to help you reprogramme your dominant mental attitude. So that you can not only change but change dramatically for the better and get a great deal more out of life by being able to put a great deal more into it.

methods of thinking, with new, viable, positive and creative ways of thinking. It shows you how to go into the flow of life once more and, more importantly, it shows you how to become creative.

The purpose of the flow programme is to help people to change their dominant mental attitude in order to help them change the direction and purpose of their lives (and thus become more creative and useful again).

As I've said earlier this is a very difficult process at first and takes at least a month of careful attention to each of the scripts on the cassettes before it gets underway.

For me it served as the aid memoir that I needed to carry me through those first few dark days of doubt and negativity and it helped support my resolve to completely change my dominant mental attitude. To change the way that I viewed the world I then lived in.

### THE FLOW

I elected to teach myself how to go into the flow simply because I realised that when you transcend yourself, when you become involved with life at a higher level than you have before, when you elect to give more and put more into life in a hundred different ways than you had ever thought of before, then you become united with the spiritual principle of life and the life force flows through you more strongly than ever before.

Once you achieve this state of personal power it is virtually impossible to hold on to any illness and you become well and happy no matter what your physical circumstances (or financial well-being).

### FINAL PRACTICALITIES

Illness, especially potentially terminal illness, is a lonely and frightening business. Probably for the first time in your life you have to confront your own mortality. You become afraid and fear freezes up your intellect so that it's difficult to think straight. You need reassurance and comfort and will take it in any form that you can get it. You will want to believe and cling to any hope or chance that some miracle will happen and you'll get better and put all this behind you.

I'm really sorry to have to tell you this but it doesn't work that way! You either take control and make up your mind once and for all to sort yourself out and get better, or you slide into dependence and the twilight of your life.

If you fear then everyone around you will pick up on that and mirror it, if you are "brave in the face of adversity" that too will be seen for the sham it is and you will evoke "admiration and sympathy" from people around you who know no other response to that stimuli.

You must step back from emotion and look at yourself and your life with the cold hard appraisal of intellect alone.

Find out and fix on what it is that has made you ill and stop doing it! Change!

Begin now ...

## BIBLIOGRAPHY

*The Vortex of Life* (nature's patterns in space and time) by Lawrence Edwards and published by Floris Books 15 Harrison Gardens Edinburgh EH11 1SH Great Britain.

*Mind Body and Electromagnetism* (Eastern and Western science fields and vibrations growth and form) by John Edwards. Published in Great Britain in 1986 by Element Books Limited.

*Electromagnetic Man* (health and hazard in the electrical environment) by Cyril W. Smith and Simon Best. Published by J.M. Dent and Sons Limited, London.

*The Water Wizard* (the extraordinary properties of natural water) by Victor Schauberger. Translated and edited by Callum Coates. Published by Gateway Books, The Hollies Wellow, Bath BA2 8QJ, UK.

*Living Energies* (an exposition of concepts related to the theories of Victor Schauberger) by Callum Coates. Gateway Books, The Hollies Wellow, Bath, BA2 8QJ UK.

*The Dark Side of the Brain* (major discoveries in the use of Kirlian Photography and electro-crystal therapy) by Harry Oldfield and Roger Coghill and published by Element Books.

*Food Enzymes* (the missing link to radiant health) by Humbart Santillo MH&ND. Published by Hohm Press, Presscot, Arizona.

*Electro-Pollution* (how to protect yourself against it) by Roger Coghill and published by Thorsons.

*Be Your Own Doctor* (a positive guide to natural living) by Anne Wigmore and published by the Avery Publishing Group, Wayne, New Jersey.

*A New Science of Life* (the hypotheses of formative causation) by Rupert Sheldrake and published by Paladin.

*Intestinal Fitness* (new light on constipation) by C. Lesley Thompson. Thorsons publishers.

*The Ghost of 29 Megacycles* (a new breakthrough in life after death) by John G. Fuller and published by Grafton Books.

*Water Electricity and Health* by Allen Hall. Published by The Hawthorne Press, Stroud, Gloucestershire.

*The Vitamin C Connection* (getting well and staying well with vitamin C) by Doctor Emanuel Cheraskin, Doctor W. Marshall Ringsdorf (Junior) and Doctor Emily L. Sisley. Published by Thorsons.

*Cancer and Vitamin C* (a discussion of the nature, causes, prevention and treatment of cancer with special reference to the value of vitamin C) by Ewen Cameron and Linus Pauling. Published by Warner Books.

*Vitamin C Against Cancer* (a medical nutritionist reports the latest findings about vitamin C as a promising new weapon in the battle against cancer — not only for treatment but for prevention) by H.L. Newbold M.D. and published by Scarborough House.

*Biologically Closed Electric Circuits* (clinical, experimental and theoretical evidence for an additional circulatory system) by Professor Bjørn E W Nordenstroøm and published by Nordic Medical Publications.

*The Power of Positive Thinking* by Norman Vincent Peel. Published by Cedar.

*Creative Visualisation* by Shakti Gawain. Published by Bantum New Age Books.

*The Mechanism of The Mind* by Doctor Malcolm Sargeant. Published by Pann Books.

*How To Make Friends and Influence People* by Dale Carnegie. Published by Cedar Books.

*The Causes and Prevention of Cancer* by Doctor Frederick B. Levenson. Published by Sidgwick and Jackson Limited, 1 Tavistock Chambers, Bloomsbury Way, London WC1A 2SG.

*The Ion Effect* by Frederick B. Soyka. Published by Bantam Books Inc, 666 Fifth Avenue N.Y. New York 10019.

## PRODUCT INDEX

The progenitor electron generator is available at a cost of £300 a unit through Sagax Publishing, 47 Haymill Close, Greenford, Middlesex, UB6 8HL.

When ordering please state the mains voltage on which you will be using this device. (This has been thoroughly tested and passed to EC safety standards and has been the subject of an interesting study at the Atomic Energy Authority a copy of which will be sent with each machine).

All orders for Progenitors will be despatched by surface mail since it weighs several kilos and will be charged at a rate of £15.00 per unit postage and packing.

The vortex unit is available at a price of £50.00 plus £5.00 postage and package from the Live Water Trust, c/o Sagax Publishing, 47 Haymill Close, Greenford, Middlesex, UB6 8HL.

The water spiraliser is available from Aquarian Angel Services, 23 West Mount, The Mount, Guildford GU2 5HL (telephone and fax 01483 572688). Costs £7.00.

Although I haven't mentioned it in the book I found Kombutcha Tea particularly helpful as I began to expand my diet and if you want to try this miracle fungus then write to the Kombutcha Network, P.O. Box 1187, Bath BA2 8YA (please send a stamped addressed envelope).

If you live in the USA then you can obtain this information from Lee Vinocur, P.O. Box 81, Palm Springs, CA92258 (telephone and fax 619 329 98